Recent Updates in Intensive Care Medicine

Edited by Nissar Shaikh

Published in London, United Kingdom

Recent Updates in Intensive Care Medicine
http://dx.doi.org/10.5772/intechopen.1000425
Edited by Nissar Shaikh

Contributors
Abdul Moeed, Abdulnasser Thabet, Ali Ayyad, Andrew Strike, Arshad Ali, Asma Batool Zaidi, De-Joseph Mibi Kakisingi, Dhaval Patel, Fizzah Batool, Germán Antonio Aguirre Gómez, Ghanem Al-sulaiti, José Antonio Villalobos Silva, Mainak Majumdar, Moyan Sun, Muhammad Arsalan Jamil, Nissar Shaikh, Obed Isaí Aguilera Olvera, Salim Surani, Sandus Khan, Schaza Javed Rana, Wael Khalaf, Zoha Bilal

First published in London, United Kingdom, 2024 by IntechOpen
IntechOpen is the global imprint of INTECHOPEN LIMITED, registered in England and Wales, registration number: 11086078, 167-169 Great Portland Street, London, W1W 5PF, United Kingdom

British Library Cataloguing-in-Publication Data
A catalogue record for this book is available from the British Library

Additional hard and PDF copies can be obtained from orders@intechopen.com

Recent Updates in Intensive Care Medicine
Edited by Nissar Shaikh
p. cm.
Print ISBN 978-0-85466-851-9
Online ISBN 978-0-85466-850-2
eBook (PDF) ISBN 978-0-85466-852-6

Meet the editor

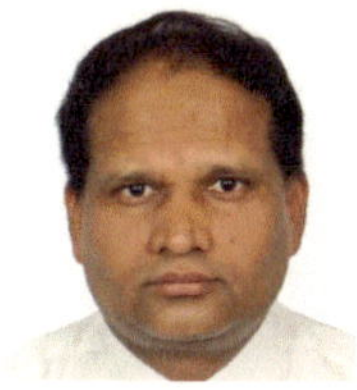

Dr. Nissar Shaikh, MD, EDIC, DID, FCCM, is a senior intensive care consultant and surgical intensive care fellowship director at Hamad Medical Corporation, Qatar. He is an associate professor at Qatar University College of Medicine and assistant professor at Weill Cornell Medicine–Qatar and an associate professor at the College of Medicine, Qatar University. Dr. Nissar has made numerous oral and poster presentations at national and international conferences. He has 200 peer-reviewed publications in critical and acute care to his credit as well as four books and 34 book chapters. He has won three prestigious awards for distinguished services from Hamad Medical Corporation.

Contents

Preface

Recent Updates in Intensive Care Medicine comprises chapters directly related to the daily practice of critical care, written by experts from various specialties and clinical environments. The content is presented in simple, accessible language, ensuring that it will not only update and assist critical care physicians but also prove invaluable to acute care physicians, surgeons, general practitioners, as well as paramedical staff and technicians working in critical, intensive, and acute care settings.

I am deeply grateful to all the contributing authors for their dedication and patience in the writing process. My heartfelt thanks go to my wife, Dr. Firdous, and my daughters, Dr. Amara and Dr. Jaza, for their unwavering support and encouragement.

Dr Nissar Shaikh MD, DiD, EDIC, FCCM
Senior Consultant SICU,
Hamad Medical Corporation,
Doha, Qatar

Associate Professor,
College of Medicine,
Qatar University,
Doha, Qatar

Assistant Professor,
Weill Cornell Medical College,
Doha, Qatar

Chapter 1

Intensive Care of Aneurysmal Subarachnoid Hemorrhage: An Update

Nissar Shaikh, Wael Khalaf, Arshad Ali, Abdulnasser Thabet, Ghanem Al-sulaiti and Ali Ayyad

Abstract

Despite the progress made in the diagnosis and management of aneurysmal subarachnoid hemorrhage (aSAH), it has remained a potentially life-threatening disease, with loss of productivity leading to social and financial losses. The recent development in diagnosis and intensive care therapy has decreased the fatality from aSAH. The Ottawa subarachnoid hemorrhage (SAH) criteria are extremely beneficial in detecting and distinguishing SAH from other causes of headaches. Furthermore, a computerized cerebral angiogram (CTA) diagnoses aSAH with high sensitivity and specificity. The Digital Subtraction Angiography (DSA) gives more accuracy about the morphology and orientation of the cerebral aneurysms. The severity of aSAH is assessed with various scores and the most frequently used one is the World Federation of Neurosurgeons Score (WFNS). The Early Brain Injury (EBI) from a ruptured cerebral aneurysm leads to raised Intracranial Pressure (ICP), hydrocephalus and/or seizures. The systemic complications of aSAH include cardiorespiratory and hormonal dysfunctions. The recent development in the management of aSAH patients begins with controlling the headache using multimodal analgesia. Following an aSAH, there will be severe hypertension, which should be treated with short-acting antihypertensives to avoid rebleeding. The ruptured aneurysm should be repaired within 24 to 72 hours. The hydrocephalus should be managed by cerebrospinal fluid (CSF) diversion via an Extra-ventricular Drain (EVD). Witnessed seizures in aSAH patients should be treated with a short course of anticonvulsants. Delayed Cerebral Ischemia (DCI) should be prevented and minimized. More recently, the cerebral vasospasm can be detected by daily Transcranial Doppler (TCD), continuous electroencephalography (cEEG), CTA, and DSA. Prompt management of cerebral vasospasm by inducing hypertension, euvolemia, and keeping serum sodium at the high-normal range is essential for minimizing the occurrence of DCI. The cerebral vasospasm resistance to this therapy is increasingly treated with chemical or balloon-assisted cerebral angioplasty. Cardiac complications in aSAH patients range from arrhythmias to acute myocardial infarction, are diagnosed early by continuous monitoring, a series of ECGs, and cardiac biomarkers, and are treated immediately. The respiratory complications in aSAH include neurogenic pulmonary edema, aspiration, ventilator-associated pneumonia (VAP), and acute respiratory distress syndrome

IntechOpen

(ARDS). These should be treated with diuretics, inotropes, early intubation, a VAP prevention bundle, and lung protective ventilation. The electrolyte disturbance and metabolic complications of aSAH such as fever, hyperglycemia, and hyponatremia are detected early with intensive care therapy and managed accordingly. Early mechanical thromboprophylaxis with the addition of pharmacological prophylaxis as soon as the aneurysm is secured has led to a significant decrease in the incidence of deep vein thrombosis as well as pulmonary embolism.

Keywords: aneurysmal subarachnoid hemorrhage, headache, hypertension, delayed cerebral ischemia, cardiorespiratory complications, euvolemia early cerebral injury, hyponatremia, hyperglycemia, hydrocephalus, intracranial pressure, seizures, vasospasm

1. Introduction

Aneurysmal subarachnoid hemorrhage (aSAH) is a severely morbid and potentially fatal condition. Prehospital mortality for aSAH patients is approximately 26%. Those who are discharged from the hospital often require rehabilitation and are generally unable to return to work. One-third of these patients need full functional support, imposing significant financial and medical burdens. The incidence of aSAH globally is around 6.1 per 100,000 per year, with Japan experiencing a higher rate of 26 per 100,000 per year [1].

Over the past three decades, the global fatality rate of aSAH has decreased by 17–50% due to advancements in ambulance services, diagnostic technologies, surgical techniques, and intensive care therapies. Equal contributions to this reduction have come from improved management of hypertension, smoking prevention, and regularly updated guidelines for aSAH management [2]. Despite the decreasing trend in aSAH incidence, an aging population and an increasing prevalence of comorbidities that elevate the risk of developing aSAH necessitate that the management team remains current with best practices to improve patient outcomes [2].

Unruptured cerebral aneurysms are increasingly detected incidentally, due to the widespread use of imaging studies [3]. Frequently, these aneurysms are small, saccular, and never rupture and their management remains controversial. The incidental unruptured fusiform, dissecting, mycotic, or traumatic aneurysm requires interventions [3]. More details on this topic will be written in a separate chapter.

2. Diagnosis of aSAH

In awake patients, the classic presentation of aSAH is a severe thunderclap headache, often described as the worst headache of their life. This headache typically peaks quickly, persists, and may be associated with nausea, vomiting, general weakness, photophobia, and neck pain or stiffness. It is crucial not to overlook the suspicion of aSAH in these patients, as emergency departments receive a significant number of headache complaints daily. Although only 3% of these cases are due to aSAH, missing this diagnosis can result in patients returning with severe disease and poor outcomes, hence the term "sentinel headache" [4].

The Ottawa subarachnoid hemorrhage rules have recently been found useful for diagnosing lower-grade aSAH patients. These criteria include signs and symptoms beyond severe headache, such as age ≥ 40 years, neck pain or stiffness, witnessed loss of consciousness, headache onset during or after exertion, and restricted neck flexion. The Ottawa SAH rules are highly sensitive (100%) but have a lower specificity of around 13%. These rules have been validated by prospective randomized studies [5].

A high-quality CT (computed tomography) scanner can detect SAH with a sensitivity of 98.7% and a specificity of 99.9% when interpreted by qualified imaging experts [6]. Thus, a negative CT brain scan performed within six hours of headache onset is likely to miss less than 1.5% of SAH cases. For the minority of CT-negative SAH cases, xanthochromia on lumbar puncture is diagnostic, with 100% sensitivity and 95.2% specificity [7].

Furthermore, computed tomographic angiography (CTA) is an important tool in the diagnosis of aSAH. CTA can differentiate between patterns of hemorrhage, such as diffuse bleeding in the basal cisterns and Sylvian fissure versus small-volume focal cortical SAH. In patients with diffuse SAH, it is recommended to perform digital subtraction angiography (DSA) to locate smaller aneurysms or vascular lesions that might escape detection due to the spatial resolution limitations of CTA [8]. DSA is the gold standard for detecting cerebral aneurysms and understanding aneurysmal geometry and cerebrovascular anatomy, which dictate treatment modalities for the aneurysms.

3. The comorbidities and risk for aSAH

The presence of various congenital and acquired comorbidities increases the risk of developing aSAH. Familial predisposition, female gender, and congenital diseases such as polycystic kidney disease and Ehlers-Danlos syndrome are significant risk factors. Modifiable risk factors include hypertension and tobacco use. Hypertension increases the risk of developing aSAH by 2.5 times, while alcohol consumption exceeding 150 grams per week doubles the risk. Non-white ethnicity is associated with a 3.4-fold increased risk of aSAH. Conversely, a lean body mass index (BMI) and hypercholesterolemia decrease the risk by 70 and 40%, respectively [9].

4. Severity scales for aSAH

The severity of aneurysmal subarachnoid hemorrhage (aSAH) is assessed using various scoring systems based on the Glasgow Coma Scale (GCS), the distribution of hemorrhage on CT brain imaging, and the presence of motor deficits. The most used severity score for aSAH is the World Federation of Neurosurgical Societies (WFNS) score. This score ranges from 0 to 5, with higher scores indicating greater severity, and incorporates the GCS and the presence or absence of motor deficits. The Hunt and Hess (H&H) score has been used for decades to evaluate aSAH severity. It also ranges from 0 to 5, based on neurological signs and symptoms, from mild headache to coma. The Fisher and modified Fisher grading systems assess aSAH severity based on the presence of hemorrhage in the subarachnoid, intraventricular, and parenchymal regions of the brain. Additionally, the Subarachnoid Hemorrhage Early Brain Edema Score (SEBES) detects global brain edema in aSAH patients and correlates well with patient outcomes [10].

5. Pathophysiology, local and systemic complication of aSAH

The sudden rupture of a cerebral aneurysm causes blood to spread into the subarachnoid space, which may extend into the ventricles and parenchyma of the brain (**Figure 1**). This leads to increased intracerebral pressure; in extreme cases, severely elevated intracerebral pressure can halt blood circulation in the brain, resulting in death.

The spillage of blood in the subarachnoid space in aSAH causes not only local cerebral complications but also systemic problems. Local cerebral injury can be early or delayed and is due to disruption of the blood–brain barrier (BBB), the release of proinflammatory cytokines and mediators, and oxidative stress, leading to cerebral microcirculatory dysfunction. These local cerebral injuries result in the development of hydrocephalus and vasospasm, causing seizure activity and hyperthermia. Together, these changes can complicate into delayed cerebral ischemia and poor prognosis.

Systemic complications after aSAH are due to autonomic nervous system, metabolic, or hormonal disturbances. Cardiac adverse effects in aSAH patients are mainly due to a surge in sympathetic and parasympathetic activity, ranging from arrhythmias to stress cardiomyopathy and neurogenic pulmonary edema. Metabolic disturbances can cause hyperglycemia. Hormonal changes may lead to the syndrome of inappropriate antidiuretic hormone (SIADH) and cerebral salt wasting syndrome (CSWS), causing hyponatremia (**Figure 1**).

6. Intensive care therapy of aSAH patients

Patients with aSAH should be admitted to and managed in the intensive care unit (ICU), where they can receive appropriate monitoring and therapy tailored to their presentation, severity, and any local or systemic complications.

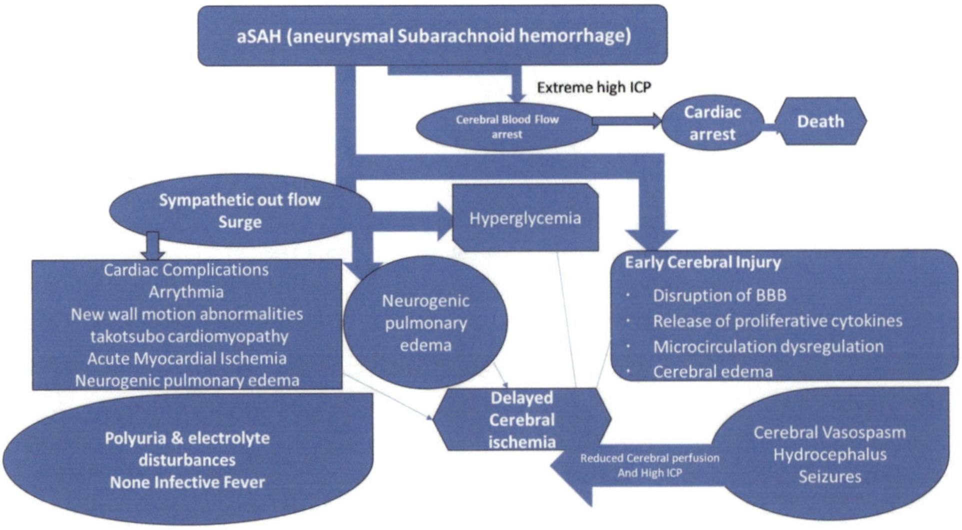

Figure 1.
Pathophysiology, local and systemic complication of aSAH.

All aSAH patients require adequate analgesia, hydration, and prophylaxis against gastric ulcers. Given the severity and multifactorial nature of their headaches, effective pain control is paramount [11]. Multimodal analgesia is recommended [11], with our practice typically initiating therapy with regular paracetamol and fentanyl as needed. Ketorolac or dihydrocodeine may be added if pain persists, and in select cases, transitioning to fentanyl patient-controlled analgesia (PCA) alongside regular paracetamol may be warranted. Dexamethasone can be introduced at any stage, typically at a dosage of 4 mg twice daily [11]. The figure illustrates our approach to analgesia in aSAH patients. We follow the Doha protocol for analgesia in aSAH patients (**Figure 2**).

Given the potential for restlessness in patients with aSAH, necessitating sedation, we have found success using dexmedetomidine at a dosage ranging from 0.7 to 1.4 mcg/kg/hour. Dexmedetomidine offers advantages over benzodiazepines, particularly in facilitating the assessment of consciousness levels.

aSAH patients often present with elevated blood pressure, a significant risk factor for rebleeding. Conversely, hypotension increases the risk of cerebral vasospasm. Therefore, it is crucial to maintain blood pressure within a target range, typically around 140 mmHg systolic, using shorter-acting antihypertensives such as labetalol or clevidipine.

Early intervention to secure the cerebral aneurysm is paramount to prevent rebleeding. It is recommended to perform aneurysm coiling or clipping within 24 to 72 hours of the ictus [12].

Antifibrinolytic agents can help stabilize clots and prevent rebleeding, but their prolonged use may elevate the risk of delayed cerebral ischemia. Therefore, their use should be judicious [13].

Hydrocephalus following aSAH can be of various types (communicating or non-communicating) and may occur acutely, sub-acutely, or chronically [14]. Acute hydrocephalus requires immediate intervention, often through external ventricular drain (EVD) insertion, lumbar drainage, or ventriculostomy, to prevent and treat

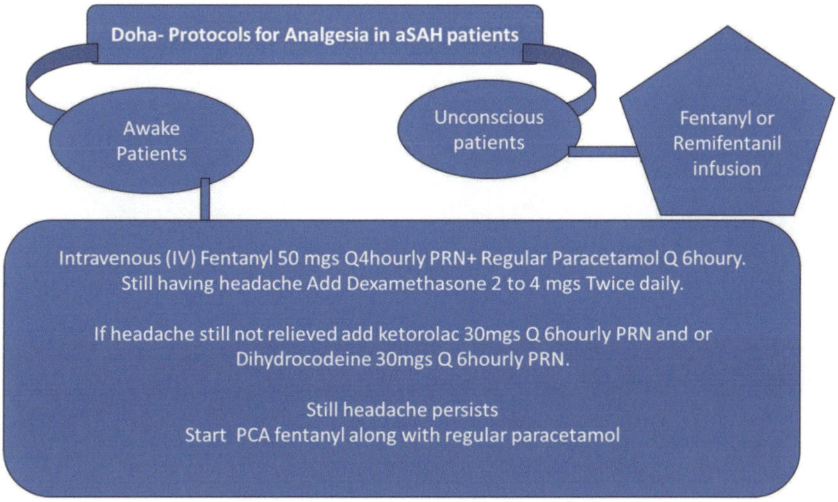

Figure 2.
Doha protocol for analgesia in aSAH.

increased intracranial pressure. Chronic hydrocephalus may necessitate the placement of a ventriculoperitoneal (VP) shunt. Care must be taken during lumbar drainage to avoid excessive cerebrospinal fluid drainage.

DCI is a concerning complication occurring in approximately 30% of patients with aSAH. Its etiology lies in cerebral vasospasm, triggered by the presence of blood and blood products surrounding cerebral vessels. Risk factors for cerebral vasospasm include female gender, smoking, hydrocephalus, hyperglycemia, and poor grade aSAH [14, 15].

Interestingly, only half of patients with angiographic vasospasm develop DCI. Moreover, DCI can occur even with a normal cerebral angiogram, as smaller vessels with spasm may evade angiographic detection. Strategies to reduce DCI risk involve oral or enteral nimodipine, along with avoiding hypovolemia and hypotension [16].

Early detection, prevention, and treatment of cerebral vasospasm before it progresses to DCI are crucial. Neurological assessments, while important, may miss DCI diagnoses. Therefore, alongside clinical monitoring, imaging studies such as transcranial Doppler (TCD), computerized cerebral angiography (CTA), or digital subtraction angiography (DSA) play significant roles. TCD, though non-invasive and bedside-compatible, has lower sensitivity compared to CTA and poorly correlates with it [17]. Continuous electroencephalography (cEEG) monitoring with analysis aids in earlier DCI detection. Combining TCD with cEEG enhances DCI diagnostic accuracy [18]. Treatment aims to improve regional cerebral perfusion and prevent DCI development. Inducing hypertension is a frequently employed intervention, reported to be safe and beneficial in reducing DCI and improving clinical outcomes. However, the ideal targeted blood pressure remains debated [19].

Balloon-assisted angioplasty or chemical angioplasty with local intra-arterial vasodilators like nimodipine or milrinone are viable options when induced hypertension fails or is contraindicated [20]. Addressing hyponatremia promptly is crucial, as it is also linked to cerebral vasospasm [21].

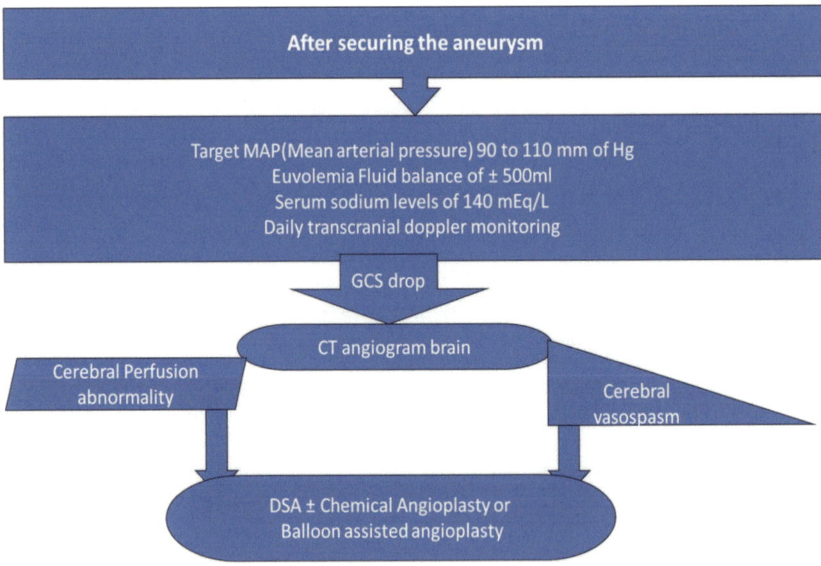

Figure 3.
Doha protocol for management of cerebral vasospasm and prevention of DCI.

To effectively prevent and manage cerebral vasospasm and DCI, we have developed and successfully implemented the Doha protocol (**Figure 3**) [22].

Seizures or status epilepticus occur in patients with aSAH, at the time of bleeding, hospitalization, or post-discharge at home. The exact etiology for convulsion in these patients is not known, it is widely believed that seizure activity occurs due to inflammation, gliosis, and cerebral hyperemia [23]. The SAFARI score is helpful in identifying the high-risk patients of aSAH for seizure activity such as the elderly, convulsions at bleed, ruptured anterior circulation aneurysms, and ventricular drainage [24]. Anticonvulsants are not indicated for routine usage in aSAH patients; however, those with aSAH deemed at high risk for developing seizures or who present with seizures or a history of convulsive activity during the bleed can be given a short course of anticonvulsants. Keppra is preferred over phenytoin due to its better pharmacokinetic and pharmacodynamic profiles. If aSAH patients develop convulsions while in hospital, this will negatively impact their prognosis.

Findings from the SYNAPSE-ICU study [25] underscore the frequent occurrence of elevated intracranial pressure (ICP) in patients with aneurysmal aSAH, often necessitating therapeutic interventions. Therefore, implementing ICP monitoring in patients with acute brain injury can significantly improve their outcomes [26].

In cases where elevated ICP leads to acute hydrocephalus, cerebrospinal fluid (CSF) drainage via diversion is the primary therapeutic approach. External ventricular drainage (EVD) stands as the gold standard for this purpose. However, the utilization of lumbar drains for CSF drainage offers a less invasive and lower infective alternative, with associated improved outcomes [26].

The risk factors predisposing aSAH patients to develop chronic hydrocephalus include higher grades, posterior circulation aneurysms, rebleeding events, higher modified Fisher scales, and multiple EVD clamping. In such cases, the treatment of choice is CSF diversion via VP shunt placement [27].

7. Extracranial complications of aSAH and their management

7.1 Cardiac complications

Cardiac complications are a significant concern for patients with aSAH, as they can complicate management and worsen prognosis [28]. These complications encompass three main types. Firstly, cardiac conduction disturbances such as sinus arrhythmias, atrial fibrillation, and ventricular tachycardia can occur, necessitating continuous electrocardiography (cECG) monitoring and frequent 12-lead ECGs [29]. Secondly, sympathetic surge-induced wall motion abnormalities may lead to heart failure with decreased cardiac output. Lastly, Takotsubo cardiomyopathy, characterized by apical ballooning of heart chambers, can develop, although it is reversible and caused by myocardial stunning [30]. Additionally, some aSAH patients may rarely experience acute myocardial infarction (AMI) [31].

7.2 Respiratory complications in aSAH and its management

Respiratory complications pose another challenge, especially for high-grade aSAH patients with low Glasgow Coma Scale (GCS) scores. They are at a heightened risk of aspiration pneumonia and ventilator-associated pneumonia (VAP) due to prolonged intubation and mechanical ventilation. Hence, strict adherence to VAP prevention bundles is essential [32]. Neurogenic pulmonary edema, affecting approximately 23% of aSAH patients, may progress to acute respiratory distress syndrome (ARDS), necessitating immediate ICP reduction and prolonged invasive ventilation [33].

Headache management Prevention of rebleed	• Multimodal analgesia • Early Securing Aneurysm • Avoid Hypertension or hypotension till aneurysm is secured
Hydrocephalus Intracranial hypertension	• Urgent External Drainage of CSF by EVD or Lumbar Drain • Intracranial Pressure Monitoring • Antiedema therapy
Seizures	• Anticonvulsant: in witnessed seizures or High-risk group patients • Consider continuous Electroencephalogram (cEEG) Monitoring and analysis
Delayed Cerebral Ischemia	• Daily Transcranial Doppler • CT Angio and perfusion studies • Chemical or mechanical Cerebral Angioplasty • Maintain Euvolemia • Serum sodium high-normal target • Induced Hypertension
Fever	• Start Therapy and temperature control management if Temperature = or > 37.5°C • Continuous Temperature Monitoring
Polyuria Hyponatremia	• Advanced hemodynamic monitoring • Optimize Hydration • Look for Cerebral Vasospasm • Frequent Electrolyte Monitoring • Maintain Serum Sodium >140 mEq/L • Fludrocortisone • Hypertonic saline
DVT Prophylaxis	• Mechanical thromboprophylaxis till the Aneurysm is secured. • Chemical thromboprophylaxis after securing aneurysm
Respiratory complications Cardiovascular complications	• Reduce intrapulmonary water • Lung protective ventilation • Ventricular Associated Bundles (VAP) bundles • Antimicrobial therapy • Continuous monitoring • Series of 12 lead ECG • POCUS and Echocardiography • Prompt diagnosis and treatment of complications

Table 1.
Summary of updated intensive care management of aSAH.

There is significant reduction in occurrence of ARDS in aSAH from 38% in 2008 to 4% in 2014 [34]. The risk of ARDS increases in aSAH patients with cerebral edema, high grades of aSAH, cardiogenic shock, and cardiac arrest. These patients need lung protective ventilation, with worse overall outcomes [35].

7.3 Metabolic disturbances in aSAH and management

Metabolic disturbances are common in aSAH patients and require careful management. Maintaining euvolemia and addressing electrolyte imbalances promptly are crucial aspects of their care. The use of albumin may maintain the intravascular volume in these patients [36]. Hyponatremia, hypokalemia, and hypophosphatemia are frequent in these patients and can cause cardiac and neurological dysfunction [16]. Hence, it is important to optimize the dyselectrolytemia quickly. The hyponatremia could be due to syndrome of inappropriate antidiuretic Hormone (SIADH) secretion, cerebral salt wasting (CSW) syndrome, or a combination of both. Prompt diagnosis and earlier management are essential [37].

Hyperglycemia, attributed to stress and hypothalamic dysfunction, requires prompt blood sugar control, balancing tight control to avoid hypoglycemia, which can be detrimental to the brain [38]. Fever is another medical complication of aSAH, and irrespective of etiology, it is associated with the worst outcome in these patients. Hence, frequent or continuous monitoring of the core body temperature and prompt control by pharmacological, mechanical, or combined therapy is essential. It is recommended to avoid a rise in temperature of more than 37.50 C [39].

7.4 Deep venous thrombosis (DVT) and pulmonary embolism (PE)

Lastly, DVT and PE are significant concerns, affecting around 20% of aSAH patients. Early mobility in awake patients and the prompt initiation of mechanical DVT prophylaxis, followed by pharmacological prophylaxis once the cerebral aneurysm is secured, are crucial to reduce morbidity and mortality associated with DVT and PE [40]. Updated Intensive care management of aSAH is summarized in **Table 1**.

8. Perioperative management of ruptured cerebral aneurysms

8.1 Preoperative evaluation

It is an emergency to secure the bleeding ruptured aneurysm, hence, the pre-anesthetic evaluation should facilitate the early surgical intervention. Apart from all demographics, clinical, and laboratory evaluations, one must mention the severity of aSAH by documenting the grade of SAH (WFNS and H&H scores) and the location of the aneurysm, as the higher grade and posterior circulation aneurysm has higher cardiorespiratory, metabolic complications and electrolyte disturbances, requiring advance hemodynamic monitoring and frequent therapeutic interventions [41].

8.2 Anesthetic management

The aim of anesthetic management of ruptured aneurysm cases is to prevent rebleeding, optimize cerebral perfusion, relax the brain, prevent edema, facilitate temporary clipping, and maintain hemodynamic stability [42]. During the induction of anesthesia, prevention of hypo- as well as hypertension is essential, as hypertension increases the risk of rebleeding by increasing the transmural pressure in the aneurysm. Hypotension can potentiate the adverse effects of temporary clipping and have an impact on cerebral ischemia. One should maintain normocarbia, as both hyper- and hypocarbia have adversely affect the brain [42]. An invasive blood pressure monitoring with the arterial line will help in preventing or minimizing the above-mentioned complications and help in frequent blood sampling. Maintenance of anesthesia can be done by total intravenous anesthesia (TIVA) or by volatile anesthetic agents. Each of these has advantages and disadvantages, recent trends are toward using the TIVA. The aim of maintaining anesthesia in these patients should be to reduce the cerebral metabolic rate, reduce or prevent intracranial hypertension, provide neuroprotection, facilitate titration and maintenance of anesthesia depth, and ensure hemodynamic stability [42]. It is common practice to induced hypertension during the temporary clipping to reduce the ischemic effects by more perfusion through the collaterals. The burst suppression is achieved with the extra dosage of various anesthetic agents, but the major issue with this is the hypotension and one must be careful [43]. Adenosine-induced temporary flow arrest is also used in complex, difficult ruptured aneurysmal surgeries, in patients without cardiac comorbidity or complications. The use of adenosine-induced flow arrest needs experience and better communication between surgeons and anesthesiologists [44].

8.3 Post-anesthesia care

The emergence from anesthesia should be smooth. Pain should be controlled by multimodal analgesia. Postoperatively, these patients should be admitted to intensive care therapy unit for frequent blood sampling and acute management of the metabolic and electrolyte disturbances. Post-cerebral aneurysm surgery, the hemodynamic management and optimization of preload by dynamic preload parameters such as stroke volume variation (SVV) and Global end-diastolic volume index (GEVI) have been shown to improve outcomes in higher grade aSAH patients. Induced hypertension, euvolemia along with higher normal serum sodium levels ara proposed in prevention of acute and delayed cerebral ischemia [45].

9. Conclusion

A ruptured cerebral aneurysm is the primary cause of spontaneous subarachnoid hemorrhage. While the fatality rate of aSAH has decreased over the past three decades, it remains a serious condition with high morbidity and mortality. The Ottawa SAH rules aid in suspecting and diagnosing aSAH, potentially preventing sentinel bleeds. Early local cerebral complications of aSAH include brain edema, seizures, hydrocephalus, and vasospasm, all of which heighten the risk of delayed cerebral ischemia (DCI). Systemic complications arise from cardiovascular, respiratory, metabolic, and hormonal disturbances due to sympathetic outflow surge. Severe intracranial pressure (ICP) elevation following aSAH can be fatal. The Subarachnoid Hemorrhage Brain Edema Score (SEBES) aids in detecting global brain edema. Patients may develop communicating or non-communicating hydrocephalus, necessitating cerebrospinal fluid drainage via external ventricular drain (EVD) or lumbar drain. Seizure occurrence warrants short-term anticonvulsants, with seizure reoccurrence indicating a poor prognosis. The SAFARI score helps identify patients at risk for seizure activity. Early detection, prevention, and management of cerebral vasospasm are crucial to prevent or reduce DCI. Apart from clinical monitoring, daily transcranial Doppler (TCD) in combination with continuous electroencephalography (cEEG) and further evaluation with CT angiography (CTA) aids in early detection.

Treatment of cerebral vasospasm involves induced hypertension, maintaining euvolemia and serum sodium levels around 140 mEq/L. Resistant vasospasm may require chemical or mechanical angioplasty. Early detection and proper management of systemic complications are essential to mitigate adverse outcomes. Continuous or frequent core body temperature monitoring is vital due to the potential adverse impact of fever. Hyperglycemia should be managed with liberal blood sugar control, while hypo- and hyperglycemia should be avoided. Reducing the occurrence of deep vein thrombosis (DVT) or pulmonary embolism (PE) involves early mobilization of awake patients and pharmacological thromboprophylaxis once the aneurysm is secured. The incidence of acute respiratory distress syndrome (ARDS) in aSAH patients is declining, and ventilator-associated pneumonia (VAP) should be prevented using VAP prevention bundles. Continuous ECG monitoring, a series of 12-lead ECGs, and cardiac biomarkers are essential for diagnosing and managing cardiac complications in aSAH patients. Above-mentioned updated perioperative care will improve aSAH patients' management.

Author details

Nissar Shaikh[1]*, Wael Khalaf[1], Arshad Ali[2], Abdulnasser Thabet[2], Ghanem Al-sulaiti[2] and Ali Ayyad[2]

1 Surgical Intensive Care, Hamad Medical Corporation, Doha, Qatar

2 Neurosurgery Section, Department of Neurosciences, Hamad Medical Corporation, Doha, Qatar

*Address all correspondence to: nissatfirdous99@gmail.com

References

[1] Hoh BL, Ko NU, Amin-Hanjani S, Chou SH-Y, Cruz-Flores S, Dangayach NS, et al. 2023 guideline for the Management of Patients with Aneurysmal Subarachnoid Hemorrhage: A guideline from the American Heart Association/ American Stroke Association. Stroke. 2023;**54**(7):e314-e370

[2] Marazzi TBM, Mendes PV. Updates on aneurysmal subarachnoid hemorrhage: Is there anything really new? Arquivos de Neuro-Psiquiatria. 2022;**80**(5 S1):1

[3] Renowden S, Nelson R. Management of incidental unruptured intracranial aneurysms. Practical Neurology. 2020;**20**:347-355

[4] Pereira JL, de Albuquerque LA, Dellaretti M, de Carvalho GT, Vieira G Jr, Rocha MI, et al. Importance of recognizing sentinel headache. Surgical Neurology International. 2012;**3**:162

[5] Jeffrey JP, Sivilotti MLA, Sutherland J, et al. Validation of the Ottawa subarachnoid Hemorrhage rule in patients with acute headache. CMAJ. 2017;**189**:E1379-E1385

[6] Dubosh NM, Bellolio MF, Rabinstein AA, Edlow JA. Sensitivity of early brain computed tomography to exclude aneurysmal subarachnoid Hemorrhage: A systematic review and meta-analysis. Stroke. 2016;**47**(3):750-755

[7] Walton M, Hodgson R, Eastwood A, Harden M, Storey J, Hassan T, et al. Management of patients presenting to the emergency department with sudden onset severe headache: Systematic review of diagnostic accuracy studies. Emergency Medicine Journal. 2022;**39**(11):818-825

[8] Rustemi O, Alaraj A, Shakur SF, Orning JL, Du X, Aletich VA, et al. Detection of unruptured intracranial aneurysms on noninvasive imaging. Is there still a role for digital subtraction angiography? Surgical Neurology International. 2015;**6**:175

[9] Sundström J, Söderholm M, Söderberg S, Alfredsson L, Andersson M, Bellocco R, et al. Risk factors for subarachnoid haemorrhage: A nationwide cohort of 950 000 adults. International Journal of Epidemiology. 2019;**48**(6):2018-2025

[10] Jan Claassen J, Carhuapoma R, Kreiter KT, Du EY, Sander Connolly E, Mayer SA. Global cerebral Edema after subarachnoid Hemorrhage: Frequency, predictors, and impact on outcome. Stroke. 2002;**33**:1225-1232

[11] Hile GB, Cook AM. Treatment of headache in aneurysmal subarachnoid hemorrhage: Multimodal approach. Interdisciplinary Neurosurgery. 2020;**22**:100857

[12] Robba C, Busl KM, Claassen J, et al. Contemporary management of aneurysmal subarachnoid haemorrhage. An update for the intensivist. Intensive Care Medicine. 2024;**50**:646-664

[13] Germans MR, Dronkers WJ, Baharoglu MI, Post R, Verbaan D, Rinkel GJE, et al. Antifibrinolytic therapy for aneurysmal subarachnoid haemorrhage. Cochrane Database of Systematic Reviews. 2022;**11**(11):CD001245

[14] Shaikh N, Chanda A, Mohammed K, Balfaqih A, Mohsin Khan M, Nahid S, et al. Aneurysmal Subarachnoid Haemorrhage (aSAH) and Hydrocephalus: Fact and Figures

[Internet]. Frontiers in Hydrocephalus. London, UK: IntechOpen; 2023

[15] Khan MM, Shaikh N, Yousaf Z, Sultan H, Sadek G, Khan A, et al. Risk factors for cerebral vasospasm in patients with aneurysmal subarachnoid Hemorrhage: A tertiary care Center experience. Asian Journal of Neurosurgery. 2022;**17**(2):242-224

[16] Oddo M, Poole D, Helbok R, Meyfroidt G, Stocchetti N, Bouzat P, et al. Fluid therapy in neurointensive care patients: ESICM consensus and clinical practice recommendations. Intensive Care Medicine. 2018;**44**(4):449-463

[17] van der Harst JJ, Luijckx Gert-Jan R, Elting JWJ, Bokkers RPH, van den Bergh WM, Eshghi OS, et al. Transcranial Doppler versus CT-angiography for detection of cerebral vasospasm in relation to delayed cerebral ischemia after aneurysmal subarachnoid Hemorrhage: A prospective single-Center cohort study: The transcranial doppler and CT-angiography for investigating cerebral vasospasm in subarachnoid hemorrhage (TACTICS) study. Critical Care Explorations. 2019;**1**(1):e0001

[18] Gollwitzer S, Groemer T, Rampp S, Hagge M, Olmes D, Huttner HB, et al. Early prediction of delayed cerebral ischemia in subarachnoid hemorrhage based on quantitative EEG: A prospective study in adults. Clinical Neurophysiology. 2015;**126**(8):1514-1523

[19] Gathier CS, van den Bergh WM, van der Jagt M, Verweij BH, Dankbaar JW, Müller MC, et al. Induced hypertension for delayed cerebral ischemia after aneurysmal subarachnoid Hemorrhage: A randomized clinical trial. Stroke. 2018;**49**(1):76-83

[20] Vatter H, Güresir E, König R, Durner G, Kalff R, Schuss P, et al. Invasive diagnostic and therapeutic Management of Cerebral VasoSpasm after aneurysmal subarachnoid Hemorrhage (IMCVS)-a phase 2 randomized controlled trial. Journal of Clinical Medicine. 2022;**11**(20):6197

[21] Escamilla-Ocañas CE, Venkatasubba Rao CP, Bershad E, Damani R. Temporal relationship between hyponatremia and development of cerebral vasospasm in aneurysmal subarachnoid Hemorrhage patients: A retrospective observational study. Journal of Stroke and Cerebrovascular Diseases. 2020;**29**(6):104789

[22] Khan DA, Shaikh DN, Khan DM, Alkubaisi DA, Al Rumaihi DG, Al-Sulaiti DG, et al. Epidemiology of spontaneous subarachnoid hemorrhage in the state of Qatar. Qatar Medical Journal. 2020;**2020**(1):19. DOI: 10.5339/qmj.2020.19

[23] Alkhachroum A, Megjhani M, Terilli K, Rubinos C, Ford J, Wallace BK, et al. Hyperemia in subarachnoid hemorrhage patients is associated with an increased risk of seizures. Journal of Cerebral Blood Flow and Metabolism. 2020;**40**(6):1290-1299

[24] Jaja BNR, Schweizer TA, Claassen J, Le Roux P, Mayer SA, Macdonald RL, et al. The SAFARI score to assess the risk of convulsive seizure during admission for aneurysmal subarachnoid Hemorrhage. Neurosurgery. 2018;**82**(6):887-893

[25] Robba C, Graziano F, Rebora P, et al. Intracranial pressure monitoring in patients with acute brain injury in the intensive care unit (SYNAPSE-ICU): An international, prospective observational cohort study. Lancet Neurology. 2021;**20**(7):548-555

[26] Wolf S, Mielke D, Barner C, Malinova V, Kerz T, Wostrack M, et al.

Effectiveness of lumbar cerebrospinal fluid drain among patients with aneurysmal subarachnoid Hemorrhage: A randomized clinical trial. JAMA Neurology. 2023;**80**(8):833-842

[27] Wilson CD, Safavi-Abbasi S, Sun H, Kalani MY, Zhao YD, Levitt MR, et al. Meta-analysis and systematic review of risk factors for shunt dependency after aneurysmal subarachnoid hemorrhage. Journal of Neurosurgery. 2017;**126**(2):586-595

[28] Norberg E, Odenstedt-Herges H, Rydenhag B, Oras J. Impact of acute cardiac complications after subarachnoid Hemorrhage on long-term mortality and cardiovascular events. Neurocritical Care. 2018;**29**(3):404-412

[29] Simonassi F, Ball L, Badenes R, Millone M, Citerio G, Zona G, et al. Hemodynamic monitoring in patients with subarachnoid Hemorrhage: A systematic review and meta-analysis. Journal of Neurosurgical Anesthesiology. 2021;**33**(4):285-292

[30] Medina de Chazal H, Del Buono MG, Keyser-Marcus L, Ma L, Moeller FG, Berrocal D, et al. Stress cardiomyopathy diagnosis and treatment: JACC state-of-the-art review. Journal of the American College of Cardiology. 2018;**72**(16):1955-1971

[31] Cerecedo-Lopez CD, Ng I, Nguyen HB, Lai PMR, Gormley WB, Patel N, et al. Incidence and outcomes of registry-based acute myocardial infarction after aneurysmal subarachnoid Hemorrhage. Neurocritical Care. 2022;**36**(3):772-780

[32] Solenski NJ, Haley EC Jr, Kassell NF, Kongable G, Germanson T, Truskowski L, et al. Medical complications of aneurysmal subarachnoid hemorrhage: A report of the multicenter, cooperative aneurysm study. Participants of the Multicenter cooperative aneurysm study. Critical Care Medicine. 1995;**23**(6):1007-1017

[33] Wang L, Ruicheng H. Neurogenic pulmonary oedema. BMJ. 2022;**379**:e069370

[34] Veeravagu A, Chen YR, Ludwig C, Rincon F, Maltenfort M, Jallo J, et al. Acute lung injury in patients with subarachnoid hemorrhage: A nationwide inpatient sample study. World Neurosurgery. 2014;**82**(1-2):e235-e241

[35] Feldstein E, Ali S, Patel S, Raghavendran K, Martinez E, Blowes L, et al. Acute respiratory distress syndrome in patients with subarachnoid Hemorrhage: Incidence, predictive factors, and impact on mortality. Interventional Neuroradiology. 2023;**29**(2):189-195

[36] Ali A, Rajeswaran AB, Shaikh N, Al-Rumaihi G, Al-Sulaiti G. Role of albumin-induced volume expansion therapy for cerebral vasospasm in aneurysmal subarachnoid hemorrhage: A systematic review. The Journal of Neurosciences in Rural Practice. 2023;**14**(4):582-590

[37] Kieninger M, Kerscher C, Bründl E, Bele S, Proescholdt M, Zeman F, et al. Acute hyponatremia after aneurysmal subarachnoid hemorrhage: Frequency, treatment, and outcome. Journal of Clinical Neuroscience. 2021;**88**:237-242

[38] Kruyt ND, Biessels GJ, DeVries JH, Luitse MJ, Vermeulen M, Rinkel GJ, et al. Hyperglycemia in aneurysmal subarachnoid hemorrhage: A potentially modifiable risk factor for poor outcome. Journal of Cerebral Blood Flow and Metabolism. 2010;**30**(9):1577-1587

[39] Lavinio A, Andrzejowski J, Antonopoulou I, Coles J, Geoghegan P, Gibson K, et al. Targeted temperature management in patients with intracerebral haemorrhage, subarachnoid haemorrhage, or acute ischaemic stroke: Updated consensus guideline recommendations by the neuroprotective therapy consensus review (NTCR) group. British Journal of Anaesthesia. 2023;**131**(2):294-301

[40] Kilgore CB, Nair SK, Ran KR, Caplan JM, Jackson CM, Fernando Gonzalez L, et al. Venous thrombo-embolism in aneurysmal subarachnoid hemorrhage: Risk factors and timing of chemoprophylaxis. Clinical Neurology and Neurosurgery. 2023;**231**:107822

[41] Chen WL, Huang CH, Chen JH, et al. ECG monitoring predicts pulmonary edema in patients with subarachnoid haemorrhage. The American Journal of Emergency Medicine. 2016;**34**:79-82

[42] Sharma D. Perioperative management of aneurysmal subarachnoid hemorrhage: A narrative review. Anaesthesiology. 2022;**133**:183-1305

[43] Shapiro BM, Wending WW, Ammaturo FJ, et al. Vascular effects of etomidate administered for electroencephalographic burst suppression in humans. The Journal of Neurosurgical Anesthesiology. 1998;**10**:231-236

[44] Vealy R, Khot A, Bendok BR. Multiple dose adenosine used to facilitate microsurgical clipping of cerebral aneurysm complicated by intraoperative rupture. A Case Report. 2017;**8**:109-112

[45] Tagami T, Kuwamoto K, Watanabe A, et al. Optimal range of global end diastolic volume for the fluid management after aneurysmal subarachnoid hemorrhage: A multicentre prospective cohort study. Critical Care Medicine. 2014;**42**:1348-1356

Chapter 2

Resuscitation in Obstetric Hemorrhage: "Less Is More"

José Antonio Villalobos Silva, Obed Isaí Aguilera Olvera and Germán Antonio Aguirre Gómez

Abstract

Obstetric hemorrhage accounts for one-third of maternal deaths worldwide. Risk factors have been identified, being common in developing countries. Mortality due to this complication has increased in recent years in countries like United States. Therefore, intensivists should be aware of the clinical tools and technology available for diagnosing and treating patients with severe hemorrhage. The main goal of resuscitation is to restore tissue oxygen delivery and perform initial management with crystalloids, while evaluating perfusion windows, which has been a long-time study, followed by transfusion of blood products (if initially not available) with the aim of restoring circulating volume. In recent years, complications of a large volume of fluids during resuscitation have proved harmful, as fluid accumulation in different organs such as the brain, heart, lung, and kidneys may cause edema, decreased lactate clearance, oxygen diffusion, weaning failure, increased hospital stay, and coagulopathy. The "less is more" approach is a strategy based on optimizing resources such as time to evaluation, treatment with fluids and blood products, clinical and laboratory data to assess severity to provide stabilization, and avoiding common complications in the ICU due to severe hemorrhage.

Keywords: obstetric hemorrhage, transfusion, fluid therapy, resuscitation, ICU

1. Introduction

Throughout the world, obstetric hemorrhage is one of the main causes of maternal death. However, there may be a great disparity between the prevalence of obstetric hemorrhage and its mortality in different countries due to individual implementation of preventive and preplanning measures in high-risk patients. The World Health Organization (WHO) has defined maternal death as the death of a woman during pregnancy or childbirth, or within 42 days of pregnancy termination, due to any cause related to or aggravated by pregnancy or its management.

A fourth of all maternal deaths in the world result from obstetric hemorrhage, accounting for approximately 140,000 deaths per year; the incidence of potentially deadly bleeding is 5–15% and is defined by the Royal College of Obstetrics and Gynecology (RCOG) as an estimated loss of blood of >2.5 liters or the required administration of >5 blood product units, or treatment of coagulopathy, all warranted in 3.7 of every 1000 pregnancies. Despite an observed decrease in the incidence of

IntechOpen

maternal deaths in the past few years, over half of them are still due to obstetric hemorrhage, whereby their incidence increased from 2.7 to 4.3% between 2000 and 2019 [1, 2]. As a result of this higher incidence, we analyzed the current therapeutic efforts used to improve the in-hospital response and thus decrease the hemorrhage-dependent mortality rate.

2. Definition

As of 2014, the American College of Obstetricians and Gynecologists (ACOG) published the reVITALize initiative and classically defined obstetric hemorrhage in the immediate postpartum period as blood loss above 1000 mL during vaginal delivery and/or secondary to a cesarean section. Bleeding quantification must be standardized although the exact measurement of blood loss in these procedures, and in general, is difficult to determine and usually underestimated, leading to inconsistent values; thus, a few medical centers have standardized the gravimetric method for its precise quantification in the operating room [3, 4]. Due to the frequent imprecision in blood loss calculation, the early intervention of a critical medicine specialist in the operating room is a recommended strategy, particularly if the patient shows signs of hypoperfusion and acute hemodynamic abnormalities that could lead to organ compromise.

The obstacles faced by low-income countries are clearly predictable. The lack of continuous medical education, insufficient resources, suboptimal infrastructure, and the paucity of qualified and certified personnel who can appropriately respond to an obstetric emergency are further complicated by the fact that many institutions are not supported by an immediate response team capable of following established care guidelines. In previously healthy women, severe hemorrhage may lead to a broad range of comorbidities: hemorrhagic shock, acute kidney failure, acute respiratory distress syndrome (ARDS), endocrine dysfunction, reperfusion injury,

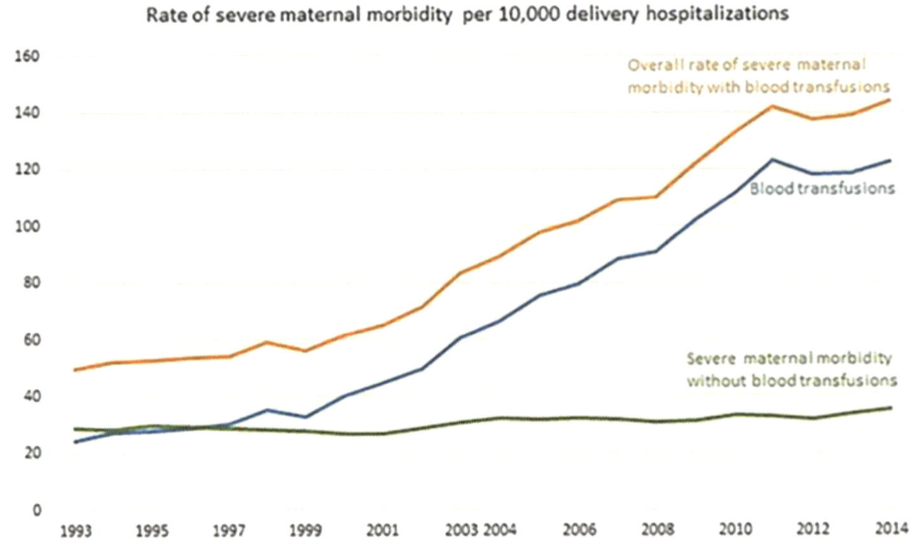

Figure 1.
Rate of severe maternal morbidity. Source: CDC.

endotheliopathy secondary to massive resuscitation, coagulopathy, etc. This is further compounded by the secondary abnormalities resulting from massive transfusion of blood products (**Figure 1**) [5, 6].

According to its temporality, obstetric hemorrhage is classified as primary if it occurs in the first 24 hours postpartum or cesarean section, and the most frequent etiology (70%) is uterine atony; less frequently, it results from placenta accreta, increta, or percreta that cause potentially deadly hemorrhages. Different studies have reported a median blood loss between 2000 and 7800 mL in placenta accreta cases (**Figure 2**). In these scenarios, resuscitation must be conservative in terms of the use of blood products, albumin, and balanced crystalloid solutions.

There are severity staging systems such as the one established by the California Department of Health that describes several stages organized according to the patient's clinical characteristics and the blood loss volume (**Figure 3**).

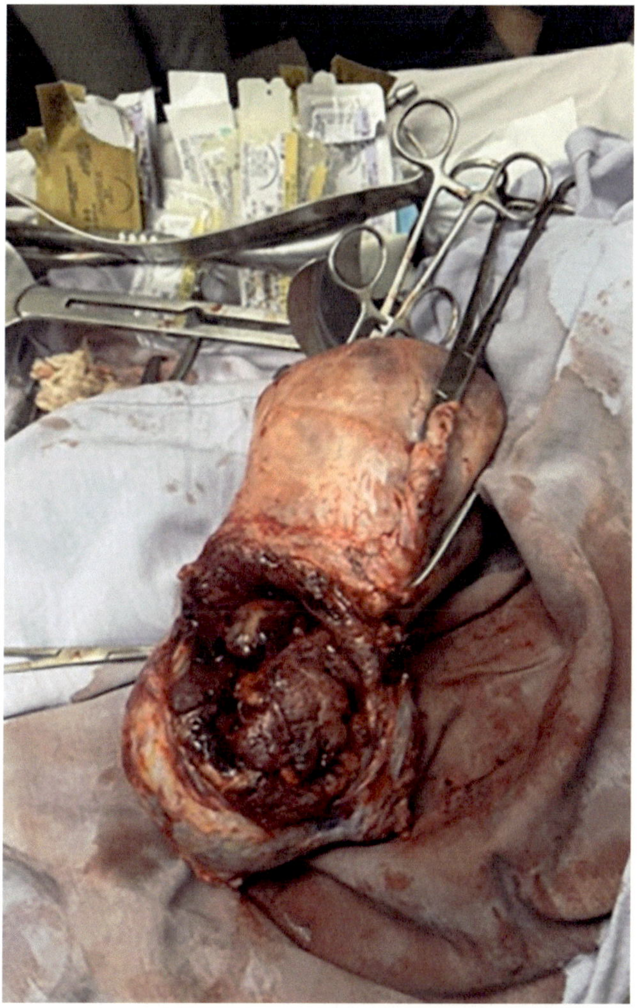

Figure 2.
Hysterectomy due to placenta percreta; hemorrhage: 7500 ml. Source: Hospital General Victoria. Tamaulipas, Mexico. 2023.

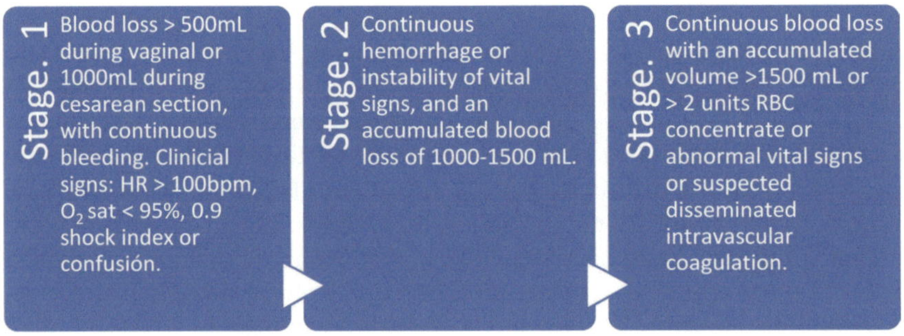

Figure 3.
The California pregnancy-associated mortality review. Report from 2002-2017 maternal death reviews. Source; Sacramento: California Department of Public Health, Maternal, Child and Adolescent Health Division, 2017.

3. Evaluation of hemorrhagic shock by the ICU team

First, one must acknowledge the available tools that can identify hemorrhage risk factors, and these have been slowly incorporated into clinical care and applied immediately before the development of hemorrhagic events (**Table 1**); identify promptly those patients at risk of warranting medical care progression if excessive hemorrhaging is observed, and obtain immediate care in the intensive care unit [8].

The early systematic evaluation of the patient in the recuperation area will reveal an obstetric patient with severe hemorrhagic shock and clinically recognizable macro- and microcirculatory findings that lead to the generation of free oxygen radicals and subsequent cell death. The patient will be at risk of multiorgan dysfunction compounded by the effects of resuscitation in the operating room resulting in ischemia-reperfusion injury and the initial phases of multiple organ dysfunction [9, 10].

Among patients at high risk of obstetric bleeding, the following parameters should be gauged before the delivery or cesarean section: metabolic status, renal function, cystatin-C, lactate, C reactive protein (CRP), coagulation profile, and acid-base status. The well-known hemodynamic changes of pregnancy include a 30–40% increase

Intermediate risk	High risk
Blood loss: 500–1000 mL	Accumulated blood loss >1000 ml
Vaginal deliveries: > 4	Placental abruption and/or active bleeding
Platelets: 50,000–100,000	Platelets: < 50,000
Hematocrit: < 30% (Hb < 10gr/dL)	Hematocrit: < 24% (< 8gr/dL)
Genital laceration (3rd–4th degree)	Known associated coagulopathy
Multiple gestations	Placenta accreta
Chorioamnionitis	HELLP

***Table 1** Adapted and used with permission from Lagrew et al., and originally adapted from the "Improving Health Care Response to Obstetric Hemorrhage: A California Quality Improvement Toolkit", funded by the California Department of Public Health, 2015; supported by Title V funds. Adaptations are also works protected by copyright. To publish this adaptation, authorization must be obtained both from the owner of the copyright of the original work and from the owner of the translation or adaptation copyright [7].*

Table 1.
Risk factors for obstetric hemorrhage.

in cardiac output (CO), systolic volume (SV) (30–40%), left ventricular ejection fraction (LVEF) (5%), and a 20–30% decrease in peripheral vascular resistance (PVR), all to increase oxygen availability (O_2A) during gestation and satisfy the additional oxygen consumption (VO_2) of the obstetric patient.

3.1 Hemorrhage ≥1000 ml in the perioperative period

Hemorrhagic shock-induced endotheliopathy (SHINE) is fostered by an effective hypovolemic state followed by adrenal activation and a secondary massive release of catecholamines leading to dysregulated endothelial activation as well as of its glycocalyx, which in turn, activate a series of different biochemical markers such as E-selectin, intracellular adhesion molecule-1 (ICAM-1), the family of four heparan sulfate proteoglycans (Syn1–Syn4) (HSPGs), and angiopoietin (Agpt-1 and Agpt-2). Simultaneously, fibrinolysis signaling is triggered, altering the coagulation pathway, particularly the phase of "coagulation amplification," which can in turn lead to the development of uncontrolled disseminated intravascular coagulation, further complicating the baseline state of hypovolemic shock [11].

During active bleeding caused in 70% of cases by uterine atony, we must not waste time making decisions, because "less is more." We must optimize the timing of every therapeutic decision and implement efforts based on guidelines with a strong grade of clinical evidence quality (GRADE). When pharmacologic interventions do not control the bleeding rate, a surgical approach should be rapidly implemented (strong recommendation, high); compression sutures, the ligation of the uterine, iliac, or internal iliac arteries, and uterine artery embolization are effective interventions to consider; however, hysterectomy should not be delayed in patients that remain unstable due to active bleeding (strong recommendation, high) [12].

During active hemorrhage, all the initial measures implemented in the operating room by the multidisciplinary team must be reinforced, whereby two peripheral, permeable intravenous accesses must be available, an electrocardiogram should be obtained or electrocardiographic monitoring should be initiated for the timely detection of myocardial ischemia secondary to the decreased availability of oxygen, and venous and/or arterial blood gases should be obtained to determine the patient's acid-base status, as well as hematocrit and lactate levels; blood gases should be closely monitored [13].

Hemostatic resuscitation is a new concept referring to the prompt replacement of the intravascular volume with blood products and further reflects the idea of "less is more": this was concluded from the results of a systematic review of various trials that compared the administration of fresh frozen plasma (FFP), platelets, and red blood cells in 1:1:1 ratio with the practice of laboratory-guided transfusion (n = 69), early cryoprecipitate transfusion following standard practice (n = 41), and early administration of fibrinogen concentrate, in comparison with placebo (n = 45); one trial compared the effect of a 1:1:1 proportion of FFP, platelets, and red blood cells with 1:1:2 proportion in terms of mortality at 24 hours and at 30 days [n = 680]; another compared treatment with [whole blood with 24-hour blood [n = 107]; another compared the administration of FFP with red blood cells at 1:1 ratio with 1:4 ratio [n = 16]; all protocols were based on limited available evidence and did not reach a conclusion on the best approach in terms of mortality or morbidity [14].

Other authors are also investigating the predictive performance of the shock index in women with bleeding ≥1000 mL, but no significant correlation has been found, with an AUC ROC of 0.54 (95% CI: 0,47–0,61), a similar value to other vital signs [15].

If available, the coagulation model must be evaluated by thromboelastography prior to admission to the intensive care unit, to consider the early administration of tranexamic acid (TXA) or another directed pharmacologic measure. Several clinical trials, two large meta-analyses, and a randomized controlled trial revealed that 1 g TXA administered intravenously in the context of early obstetric bleeding can decrease blood loss, rate of hysterectomies, and most probably, mortality [16, 17]. A recent placebo-controlled trial revealed that the prophylactic administration of tranexamic acid during cesarean section did not decrease the risk of maternal death or the need for blood transfusions [18].

3.2 Transfer and admission to the intensive care unit (ICU)

The transfer of patients with obstetric hemorrhage must be as timely as possible once the intensive care team has evaluated the patient's status and analyzed the potential risks implicit in the transfer. In patients who are hemodynamically unstable and mechanically ventilated, in terms of timelines, again, "less is more," whereby the transfer should be prompt as the patient will require early interventions by the ICU team, such as the placement of monitoring equipment, precise and personalized adjustments to mechanical ventilation to prevent ventilator-induced lung injury (VILI), and set up an alveolar protection ventilation model [18, 19].

During the transfer to the ICU, the patient must be continuously monitored electrocardiographically as well as via pulse oximetry, her blood pressure must be periodically measured non-invasively, and the heart and respiratory rates should be easily visualized on the monitor; some selected patients may benefit from capnography. All drugs initiated before the transfer such as vasoactive, inodilator, antiarrhythmic, and/or sedating drugs must still be administered with continuous infusion pumps powered with portable batteries. All patients who require intubation and mechanical ventilation due to hemodynamic instability should be transferred with a transport ventilator, and initial ventilatory parameters should be maintained unless the ICU team decides to increase or activate the 100% oxygen in the first 2-minute function and then make further necessary adjustments [20–22].

3.3 Resuscitation in the ICU

In the presence of a massive hemorrhage that could potentially lead to hemodynamic instability and clear signs of hypoperfusion, crystalloid solutions must be combined with albumin and blood products, while still individualizing every case to prevent hemodilution, coagulopathy, and mainly, fluid retention with positive balances in the first 24 hours.

Three physiological concepts are key in a hemorrhagic shock scenario in obstetric patients: the evaluation of response to fluid administration, circulatory reserve, and microcirculation. One way to test these variables is with a fluid challenge, administering initially a balanced crystalloid solution (Ringer Lactate, Ringer Acetate, Plasma-Lyte), the most similar solution to plasma. The underlying physiological principle of this maneuver is an attempt to increase the mean systemic filling pressure (Pmsf) to increase the systemic venous return per the central venous pressure (CVP) and hence increase the cardiac output by increasing the compartment volume: the "stressed volume."

In septic shock with borderline bleeding volume, and in which hypovolemia is greater, the state of hypoperfusion and shock is secondary to a vasodilated state with relative hypovolemia; the Frank-Starling mechanism is tested and allows to determine the benefit of fluid administration for resuscitation purposes. In severe hemorrhage scenarios, the test aims to evaluate the Frank-Starling mechanism and establish whether blood loss has been physiologically stanched, whether the arteriolar system is functional or if we are faced with an uncontrollable hemorrhage.

If blood loss is severe or if consumption coagulopathy develops during the active hemorrhage, platelets must be transfused and maintained at a value $>50 \times 10^9$/L. The main purpose of fresh plasma administration is to maintain an INR <1.8; fibrinogen should always be maintained above 2 g/L, and if necessary, several cryoprecipitate units should be administered to increase its value by 150–200 mg/dL. Another option is the use of fibrinogen concentrates (RiaSTAP) at a dose of 60–70 mg/kg weight or a standard dose of 4 g, which may increase serum fibrinogen up to 100 mg/dL [23].

In animal hemorrhagic shock models, systemic endothelial inflammation is induced and increases the risk of multiple organ dysfunction. Shedding of the endothelial glycocalyx may be secondary to the activation of cell signaling; however, the therapeutic use of unbalanced crystalloid solutions may also cause this injury. Crystalloids have been one of the most studied interventions in resuscitation scenarios; the administration of this treatment modality must be thought through since sooner or later, we must face their secondary effects; their use, however, is indispensable in the initial stages of hypovolemic shock. In a hemorrhagic shock canine model, Smart et al. observed that the administration of up to 80 ml/kg of crystalloids led to a considerable increase in endothelial inflammatory markers such as interleukin-6 (IL-6), interleukin-8 (IL-8), interleukin-10 (IL-10), and hyaluronan in comparison with colloids and blood products [24].

Xavier Monnet et al. referred that resuscitation with a rapidly administered load of crystalloid fluids (250–500 ml in 10–15 minutes) in hemorrhagic shock does not increase cardiac output (CO) but rather improves tissue oxygenation albeit not constantly, even in patients who respond well to fluid administration; hence, the response tends to be dynamic and inconsistently harmful, so treatment must be personalized [25].

Despite the development of shock, and the appropriate medical management of bleeding as well as the correction of macrohemodynamic parameters with transfusions, the microvasculature frequently remains altered: a concept known as hemodynamic coherence [26].

Functional capillary density refers to the capillary segments in which a red blood cell transits in an interval of 15 seconds and, that with the venular exit, allows the performance of two relevant physiological phenomena: optimization of O_2 transport to cells by convection and diffusion, important markers of microvascular perfusion that are key to maintain the integrity of endothelial glycocalyx [27]. In other words, fluid therapy seeks to improve convection, and real hypovolemia states in the territory of functional microcirculatory hemodynamics (FMH), thus ameliorating the volume quantity transported per second in the microcirculation. Diffusion refers to the maintenance of the functional capillary density (FCD) by not excessively increasing interstitial edema due to liberal resuscitation measures and decreasing oxygen diffusion from the capillaries to the mitochondria (**Figure 4**).

3.4 Focusing on resuscitation in obstetric hemorrhage

The first "resuscitation" insult refers to the initial 59 minutes in which there is an imminent risk of death if the primary disorder is not corrected, such as in severe hypovolemia due to the hemorrhage. This initial phase may last 3 to 6 hours in septic

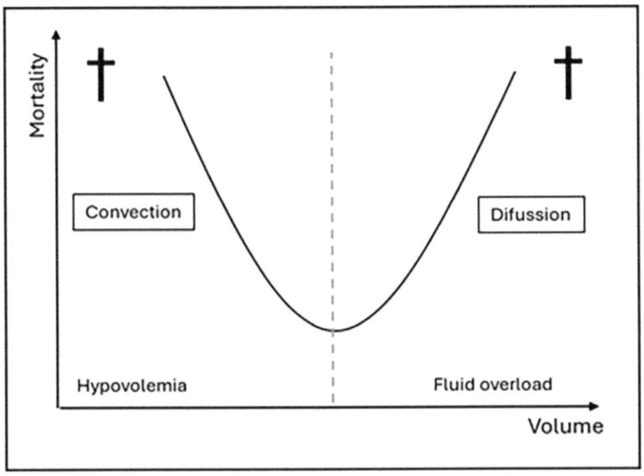

Figure 4.
Non-liberal resuscitation balance vs. early deresuscitation/de-escalation. U-shape relationship between hypovolemia/fluid overload and mortality (Adapted from Bellamy's theoretical framework) [28].

shock but is much shorter in continuous obstetric hemorrhages, which is why prompt therapeutic management is mandatory. This is the time point in which bolus fluid administration is most relevant, although this strategy should be temporary until blood products are available, so we can avoid hemodilution in a patient with an already limited circulating blood volume. It is not necessary to wait for the hemoglobin result to initiate resuscitation with intravenous fluids as it only informs us of its baseline value. The purpose of this phase is to restore the circulating volume, preserve tissue oxygenation, revert or prevent the development of coagulopathy, and eliminate/treat the underlying obstetric hemorrhage source.

"Optimization," the second phase, refers to the second insult: ischemia-reperfusion. The critical decision on when to stop fluid therapy becomes key. In the case of obstetric hemorrhages, this will occur once bleeding is under control, macro- and microcirculatory perfusion indices are adequate, and laboratory test results have been obtained (coagulogram, coagulation profile, bleeding time, viscoelastic tests, etc.).

The third phase, "stabilization," refers to the success of the previously administered therapies, and this is the point at which intravenous fluids, including solutions, and drug diluents should be strictly controlled.

Finally, the "evacuation" phase represents the evaluation of fluid accumulation due to its deleterious effects on organs such as the heart, lungs, liver, and kidneys. At this point, the intensive care physician must ask him/herself two questions: when to begin removing fluid and when to stop removing it [29–31].

As previously mentioned, the endothelial glycocalyx is the main target responding to a state of shock, in response to changes in blood flow, perfusion pressure, and blood viscosity. This is relevant because the injury caused by inflammatory mediators leads to endotheliopathy or SHINE (shock-induced endotheliopathy) that has been linked with hemostatic abnormalities, either pro or antithrombotic. Viscoelastic hemostatic tests or assays have required decades of study in coagulation disorders, particularly when applied to liver transplants and heart surgery [32]. It is not infrequent for coagulation disorders to develop in association with obstetric hemorrhage, and they are reflected in prolonged coagulation times, hypofibrinogenemia, and/or thrombocytopenia, especially in catastrophic scenarios [33].

Therefore, a disadvantage to the use of crystalloids during resuscitation is the referred endothelial glycocalyx injury, despite their low cost and availability. In hemorrhagic shock, resuscitation with fresh frozen plasma has been shown to decrease pulmonary capillary hyperpermeability and syndecan-1 levels when compared with crystalloids such as Ringer's lactate; less volume is also needed to ensure macrohemodynamic perfusion [34]. Patients in hemorrhagic shock have high levels of syndecan-1 that invariably decrease after resuscitation unlike crystalloids such as saline solution that increase endothelial permeability; hence, early administration of fresh frozen plasma is recommended [35, 36].

3.5 Coagulopathy and blood-derived products

Hemostatic viscoelastic tests were introduced as a research tool in 1948, and have been useful for several decades as a reference to the appropriate reanimation when the use of blood products is warranted. **Table 2** shows the proposed values of the various results obtained with the commercial tests, rTEG® 5000 and ROTEM® [37]. **Figure 5** presents the components of TEG®.

The use of these assays in obstetrics has been evaluated in several clinical trials and systematic reviews, particularly to predict the development of coagulopathy in patients with pre-eclampsia. Two therapeutic approaches have been evaluated in the management of obstetric hemorrhage: one in which the patient is hemodiluted (due to the use of crystalloid fluids), and the other when using blood product transfusions with viscoelastic test guidance. Despite the advantages offered by these tests such as a decreased need for blood transfusions or specific blood products if deficient, standard tests such as the prothrombin time and activated thromboplastin time remain very useful when detecting coagulation abnormalities and correlate well with blood loss. A clear disadvantage of this reanimation strategy is its complexity and the added cost of viscoelastic assays. Undeniably, viscoelastic tests are an area of opportunity in massive obstetric hemorrhage, decreasing the frequency of multiple transfusions and their known consequences [38, 39].

The management of hemorrhagic coagulopathy will depend on its phenotype or clinical presentation, manifested as either hypocoagulable or hyperfibrinolytic state,

rTEG® trigger value	ROTEM® trigger value	Intervention
ACT >128 s	EXTEM CT < 80 s	CCP/FFP
α angle <65° MAff/CFF < 11 mm	EXTEM α angle <63° FIBTEM CA 10 < 7 mm	Fibrinogen/cryoprecipitate
MA < 55 mm	MCF < 45 mm	Fibrinogen/cryoprecipitate/platelets
LY30/60 > 7.5%	EXTEM CLI30/60 < 82% ML < 15%	TXA/Aminocaproic acid

Abbreviations: Activated coagulation time (ACT); clot amplitude at 10 min (CA10); clot lysis index at 60 minutes after CT (CLI60); coagulation time (CT); extrinsic thromboelastometry activator (EXTEM); fresh frozen plasma (FFP); fibrinogen-based thromboelastometry (FIBTEM); lysis at 30 min (LY30); maximal amplitude (MA); functional fibrinogen, TEG (MAff/CFF); maximum clot firmness (MCF); prothrombin complex concentrate (PCC); maximum lysis after 30/60 min (ML30/60); rotational thromboelastometry (ROTEM®); Rapid TEG (rTEG®); Thromboelastography (TEG®); tranexamic acid (TXA) [37].

Table 2.
Proposed trigger values for rTEG® 5000 and ROTEM®.

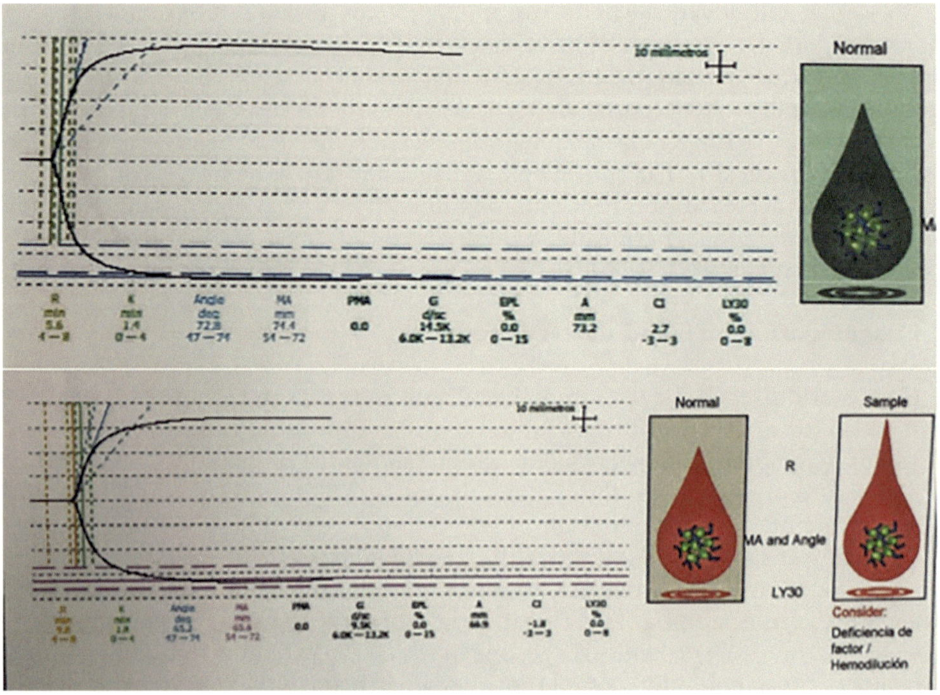

Figure 5.
TEG® of a cardiac surgery patient. Superior image shows low α-angle and maximum amplitude during active bleeding. Inferior image resulted after fresh frozen plasma and cryoprecipitate administration. Source: High Specialty Regional Hospital, Victoria, Tamaulipas, Mexico, 2023.

and the patient's status may worsen due to uncontrollable bleeding, hemodilution, and/or hypocalcemia due to products with citrate. Therefore, there are different phenotypes upon which management with blood products or anticoagulant drugs will depend [40]. Viscoelastic assays are helpful in damage control management, whereby transfusions are administered to fulfill a physiological objective. A study conducted in 2015 analyzed reanimated patients treated with cryoprecipitates to correct the fibrinogen levels before the routine availability of ROTEM in the hospital (57 patients), and after (28 patients), and showed a decreased need for transfused blood products ($p < 0.001$), less warranted hysterectomies, admissions to the ICU, and shorter hospitalization, perhaps the result of rapid correction of the coagulopathy [41]. Current evidence supports the use of transfusions based on physiological parameters in patients with massive hemorrhage [42].

The use of blood components is a complex process that requires fine tuning the risk-benefit ratio, and timely decisions decrease morbidity and mortality. The current recommendation when transfusing packed red blood cells hinges on a hemoglobin level < 7 g/dL or in the case of symptomatic active hemorrhage, 8–10 g/dL (hematocrit 21–24%), with changing values over a six-hour period. The presence of thrombocytopenia is established with platelet values below 100,000/μL; platelet administration, either concentrates or by apheresis, must be considered when values are below 50,000/μL, and bleeding is active. In vaginal deliveries, platelets should be transfused if their value is under 1000/μL. Concentrations below 10,000/μL may lead to spontaneous bleeding. The prothrombin time and the international normalized ratio (TP/INR) are used to evaluate the extrinsic pathway, and clinically, they assess fibrinogen and factor II, V, VII, and X deficiencies. The aim is to maintain the INR between 1.5 and 2. Evaluation of the intrinsic pathway is based on the activated thromboplastin time (aPTT). If the aPTT is 1.5 times above the upper normal limit, transfusion of fresh frozen plasma (FFP) should be considered. The use of fibrinogen is also important in patients in whom it has decreased 1 g/dl as they have a 2.6-fold greater risk of severe bleeding. Fibrinogen should be administered to maintain its value between 150 and 200 mg/dl [43].

The use of blood products entails risks such as transfusion reactions or the transmission of pathogens. Most reactions are considered minor and include nonhemolytic febrile reactions, hemolytic reactions, anaphylaxis, and TRALI (transfusion-related acute lung injury) or TACO (transfusion-associated circulatory overload). A clear understanding of these events and their therapeutic approach is most relevant because although transfusions are the main treatment in the reanimation of patients with obstetric hemorrhage, they may also increase the rate of complications and the duration of the in-hospital stay [44].

3.6 Deresuscitation and de-escalation

The final step in resuscitation is to deal with the consequences of the employed therapy in case large blood product and solution volumes were administered, a process known as deresuscitation. This concept describes the active removal of fluid by ultrafiltration (UF) in patients with fluid overload. As soon as resuscitation is successful, the de-escalation phase must begin, decreasing the volume of the administered solutions, be they crystalloids, blood products, or drugs, and promoting the early use of diuretics to maintain an overall balance of zero.

When the fluid balance negatively impacts an organ as in patients with difficult extubation, deresuscitation must be initiated; because of deleterious effects on organs such as the heart, lung, gastrointestinal tract, kidney, abdominal cavity, and central nervous system, several therapeutic strategies must be implemented, including the use of diuretics – loop diuretics, aldosterone antagonists, or thiazides are highly recommended [45].

In cases of resistance to diuretics, Chawla et al. have suggested using the furosemide stress test when acute kidney injury (KDIGO I-II) is suspected early in the patient's course; a dose of 1–1.5 mg/kg is administered, the response is evaluated whereby diuresis should be apparent within the following 2 hours, and the use of ultrafiltration is recommended [46].

4. Complications

The mortality resulting from continuous massive hemorrhage is the result of metabolic complications and a general state of hypoperfusion that throughout the first 24 hours may trigger irreversible coagulopathy, prolonged bleeding, and in the worst-case scenario, multiple organ dysfunction and early death. Damage-control conservative resuscitation attempts to revert organ dysfunction and avoid the trauma-lethal prognosis triad (hypothermia, acidosis, and coagulopathy) which could in turn partially or completely control hemorrhaging and preclude the development of a vicious circle in which the patient continues bleeding [47].

In obstetric hemorrhage, hypothermia is usually due to hampered cellular heat kinetics secondary to severe tissue hypoperfusion. It is usually worsened and exacerbated by intraoperative heat loss resulting from inadequate preventive maneuvers such as the lack of intraoperative heated blankets, reanimation with cold crystalloid fluids, and perhaps most importantly, prolonged exposure of the open abdominal cavity during surgery. In this setting, aside from the significant bleeding, the patient's course may be complicated by hypothermia-induced cardiac arrhythmias, a decrease in cardiac output, and an abnormal hemoglobin-oxygen dissociation curve that increases erythrocyte oxygen affinity and decreases its release into cells [48].

Metabolic acidosis, mostly resulting from anaerobic metabolism, and secondarily from increased blood lactate concentrations during obstetric bleeding, leads to a drop in intracellular and extracellular pH, which in turn causes hemodynamic failure and progressive organ and system shutdown. A pH < 7.2 worsens the cardiovascular function by increasing the amplitude of the systolic calcium transient, thus altering calcium binding to troponin C and decreasing its systolic properties [49].

Any specialist's patients may require transfusions, but obstetric hemorrhage is one of the complications that most frequently warrants massive transfusions defined as the administration of 10 units or more of whole blood or packed red blood cells over 24 hours. On rare occasions, ultramassive transfusions are needed and are defined as the need for more than 20 units of packed red blood cells over a 24–48-hour period. The main objective of a massive transfusion is to prevent the deadly results of critical complications relating to hypoperfusion while we attempt to achieve hemostasis. In the final phases, coagulopathy develops due to coagulation factor consumption and activation due to the hemorrhage per se and the administration of multiple transfusions; dilution, prolonged shock, hypoxia-induced acidosis, and hypothermia decrease the activity of coagulation factors. Another process resulting from multiple transfusions is metabolic alkalosis due to sodium citrate and citric acid in blood products. Hypocalcemia also develops as the metabolism of citrate generates 23 mEq of bicarbonate per blood unit and compromises oxygen delivery to cells. Hypocalcemia may also promote the development of arrhythmias with QT interval alterations that combined may lead to fatal outcomes [50].

Transfusion-related acute lung injury (TRALI), transfusion-related circulatory overload (TACO), and acute respiratory distress syndrome (ARDS) are characterized by pulmonary injury with accumulation of fluids in the interstitium, reflected as low- or high-pressure pulmonary edema depending on its origin. It is manifested as progressive respiratory failure with a high possibility of associated cardiopulmonary dysfunction and deadly cardiovascular outcomes. Despite the different conditions that can generate these complications, it is important to distinguish them as their etiology-directed management will lead to better results [51].

5. Conclusions

Obstetric hemorrhage is common in developing countries, accounting for less than 3% of ICU admissions. However, its social impact implies that the resources available in the critical care area are used for correct resuscitation from shock to avoid fatality. The initial approach involves clinical skills to identify signs of tissue hypoperfusion, restore cardiac output by initially administering volume, and quick and secure transport to ICU.

Detecting coagulation alterations is important because it involves identifying the blood component indicated to correct said alteration. In this way, the use of viscoelastic tests arises as an aid to limit the amount of blood products transfused, without leaving aside the usefulness of classic tests that evaluate intrinsic and extrinsic pathways. The "less is more" care strategy is aimed at optimizing the use of time and therapeutic resources and thus limiting the complications of the use of large resuscitation volumes. All these are aimed at restoring DO2, microvascular perfusion, limiting endothelial damage, and preventing and reversing coagulopathy.

It is preferable to avoid fluid accumulation due to aggressive resuscitation, although not uncommon that it occurs. Deresuscitation implies the active elimination of fluid accumulation that causes alteration in organ perfusion, increased hydrostatic capillary pressure, impaired lactate clearance, and weaning failure, mainly with drugs and ultrafiltration. This last part of critical care has an impact in improving prognosis in obstetric patients.

"Less is more" implies the knowledge of available resources to identify, resuscitate, transport, assess, and treat hemorrhagic shock in obstetric patients.

Conflict of interest

The authors declare no conflict of interest.

Author details

José Antonio Villalobos Silva*, Obed Isaí Aguilera Olvera
and Germán Antonio Aguirre Gómez
Critical Care Department, High Specialty Regional Hospital "Bicentenario 2010", Victoria, Tamaulipas, México

*Address all correspondence to: umae_abc@yahoo.com.mx

References

[1] Say L, Chou D, Gemmill A, et al. Global causes of maternal death: A WHO systematic analysis. Lancet Global Health. 2014;**2**(6):e323-e333

[2] Kassebaum NJ, Barber RM, Bhutta ZA, et al. Global, regional, and national levels of maternal mortality, 1990-2015: A systematic analysis for the global burden of disease study 2015. Lancet. 2016;**388**:1775-1812

[3] Smith CM, Borders AE, et al. ACOG Committee opinion summary 794. Quantitative blood loss in obstetric hemorrhage. Obstetrics and Gynecology. 2019;**134**:1368-1369

[4] Vitello DJ, Ripper RM, Fettiplace MR, Weinberg GL, Vitello JM. Blood density is nearly equal to water density: A validation study of the gravimetric method of measuring intraoperative blood loss. Journal of Veterinary Medicine [Internet]. 2015;**2015**:7-9. DOI: 10.1155/2015/152730

[5] Neary C, Naheed S, McLernon DJ, et al. Predicting risk of postpartum haemorrhage: A systematic review. BJOG: An International Journal of Obstetrics and Gynaecology. 2021;**128**:46-53

[6] Nathan LM. An overview of obstetric hemorrhage. In: Seminars in Perinatology. Vol. 43, No. 1. WB Saunders, Elsevier Inc.; 2019. pp. 2-4

[7] Abbas D, Wang MJ, Claus L, et al. Intrapartum risk factors and prediction of obstetric hemorrhage-related morbidity. American Journal of Perinatology. 2021. DOI: 10.1055/a-1975-4688

[8] Hacker FM, Phillips JM, Lemon LS, et al. Comparative analysis of obstetric hemorrhage risk prediction tools. American Journal of Perinatology. 2022;**40**(15):1687-1694. DOI: 10.1055/s-0041-1740013

[9] Lagrew D, McNulty J, Sakowski C, et al. Improving Health Care Response to Obstetric Hemorrhage, a California Maternal Quality Care Collaborative Toolkit. California Department of Public Health; 2022

[10] Gutierrez G, Reines HD, Wulf-Gutierrez ME. Clinical review: Hemorrhagic shock. Critical Care (London, England). 2004;**8**:373-381. DOI: 10.1186/cc2851

[11] Chouchani ET, Pell VR, James AM, Work LM, Saeb-Parsy K, Frezza C, et al. A unifying mechanism for mitochondrial superoxide production during ischemia-reperfusion injury. Cell Metabolism. 2016;**23**:254-263. DOI: 10.1016/j.cmet.2015.12.009

[12] Johansson P, Stensballe J, Ostrowski S. Shock induced endotheliopathy (SHINE) in acute critical illness - a unifying pathophysiologic mechanism. Critical Care. 2017;**21**:25. DOI: 10.1186/s13054-017-1605-5

[13] Goncharov NV, Nadeev AD, Jenkins RO, Avdonin PV. Markers and biomarkers of endothelium: When something is rotten in the state. Oxidative Medicine and Cellular Longevity. 2017;**2017**:9759735. DOI: 10.1155/2017/9759735. Epub 2017 Nov 23

[14] Robinson D, Basso M, Chan C, Duckitt K, Lett R. Guideline No. 431: Postpartum hemorrhage and hemorrhagic shock. Journal of Obstetrics and Gynaecology Canada. 2022;**44**(12):1293-1310.e1. DOI: 10.1016/j.

jogc.2022.10.002 [Erratum in: J Obstet Gynaecol Can. 2023 Mar 11: Erratum in: J Obstet Gynaecol Can. 2023 Jun 26]

[15] McQuilten ZK et al. Optimal dose, timing and ratio of blood products in massive transfusion: Results from a systematic review. Transfusion Medicine Reviews. 2018;**32**(2018):6-15

[16] Mizutani H, Ushida T, Ozeki K, et al. Predictive performance of shock index for postpartum hemorrhage during cesarean delivery. International Journal of Obstetric Anesthesia [Internet]. 2023;(November):103957. DOI: 10.1016/j.ijoa.2023.103957

[17] Brenner A, Shakur-Still H, Chaudhri R, et al. El impacto de los eventos de resultados tempranos en el efecto del ácido tranexámico en la hemorragia posparto: un análisis exploratorio del subgrupo del ensayo WOMAN. BMC Embarazo Parto. 2018;**18**:215

[18] Pacheco LD, Clifton RG, Saade GR, Weiner SJ, Parry S, Thorp JM Jr, et al. Eunice Kennedy Shriver National Institute of child health and human health and human human medicine units network. Ácido tranexámico para prevenir la hemorragia obstétrica después del parto por cesárea. The New England Journal of Medicine. 2023;**388**(15):1365-1375. DOI: 10.1056/NEJMoa2207419

[19] Sentilhes L, Senat MV, Le Lous M, et al. Ácido tranexámico para la prevención de la pérdida de sangre después del parto por cesárea. The New England Journal of Medicine. 2021;**384**:1623-1634

[20] Fanara B, Manzon C, Barbot O, Desmettre T, Capellie G. Recommendations for the intra-hospital transport of critically ill patients. Critical Care. 2010;**14**:R87

[21] Shirley PJ, Bion JF. Intra-hospital transport of critically ill patients: Minimizing risk. Intensive Care Medicine. 2004;**30**(8):1508-1510

[22] Warren J, Fromm RE, Orr RA, et al. American College of Critical Care Medicine. Guidelines for the inter- and intrahospital transport of critically ill patients. Crit Care Med. 2004;**32**(1):256-262. DOI: 10.1097/01.CCM.0000104917.39204.0A

[23] Ducloy-Bouthors AS, Mercier FJ, Grouin JM, et al. Administración temprana y sistemática dc concentrado de fibrinógeno en hemorragia posparto después del parto vaginal: el ensayo controlado aleatorizado FIDEL. BJOG. 2021;**128**:1814-1823

[24] Lumbreras-Marquez MI, Villela-Franyutti D, Reale SC, et al. Manejo de la coagulación en anestesia obstétrica. Current Anesthesiology Reports. 2022;**12**:266-276

[25] Monnet X, Malbrain MLNG, Pinsky MR. The prediction of fluid responsiveness. Intensive Care Medicine [Internet]. 2023;**49**(1):83-86. DOI: 10.1007/s00134-022-06900-0

[26] Ince C. Hemodynamic coherence and the rationale for monitoring the microcirculation. Critical Care [Internet]. 2015;**19**(Suppl. 3):S8. Available from: http://www.ccforum.com/content/19/S3/S8

[27] Smart L, Boyd CJ, Claus MA, Bosio E, Hosgood G, Raisis A. Large-volume crystalloid fluid is associated with increased hyaluronan shedding and inflammation in a canine hemorrhagic shock model. Inflammation. 2018;**41**(4):1515-1523

[28] Bellamy MC. Wet, dry or something else? British Journal of Anaesthesia

[Internet]. 2006;**97**(6):755-757. DOI: 10.1093/bja/ael290

[29] Bonanno FG. Management of hemorrhagic shock: Physiology approach, timing and strategies. Journal of Clinical Medicine. 2023;**12**(1):260

[30] Jani VP, Jani VP, Munoz CJ, Govender K, Williams AT, Cabrales P. Application of negative tissue interstitial pressure improves functional capillary density after hemorrhagic shock in the absence of volume resuscitation. Physiological Reports. 2021;**9**(5):1-12

[31] Malbrain MLNG, Van Regenmortel N, Saugel B, De Tavernier B, Van Gaal PJ, Joannes-Boyau O, et al. Principles of fluid management and stewardship in septic shock: It is time to consider the four D's and the four phases of fluid therapy. Annals of Intensive Care [Internet]. 2018;**8**(1):66. DOI: 10.1186/s13613-018-0402-x

[32] Guasch E, Gilsanz F. Massive obstetric hemorrhage: Current approach to management. Medicina Intensiva. 2016;**40**(5):298-310

[33] Faria I, Thivalapill N, Makin J, Puyana JC, Raykar N. Bleeding, hemorrhagic shock, and the global blood supply. Critical Care Clinics. 2022;**38**(4):775-793

[34] Bunch CM, Chang E, Moore EE, Moore HB, Kwaan HC, Miller JB, et al. Shock-induced endotheliopathy (SHINE): A mechanistic justification for viscoelastography-guided resuscitation of traumatic and non-traumatic shock. Frontiers in Physiology. 2023;**14**:1-34

[35] Turkoglu O, Friedman P. Evaluation during postpartum hemorrhage. Clinical Obstetrics and Gynecology. 2023;**66**(2):357-366

[36] Peng Z, Pati S, Potter D, Brown R, Holcomb JB, Grill R, et al. Fresh frozen plasma lessens pulmonary endothelial inflammation and hyperpermeability after hemorrhagic shock and is associated with loss of syndecan 1. Shock. 2013;**40**(3):195-202

[37] Volod O, Bunch CM, Zackariya N, Moore EE, Moore HB, Kwaan HC, et al. Viscoelastic hemostatic assays: A primer on legacy and new generation devices. Journal of Clinical Medicine. 2022;**11**(3):860

[38] Anand T, Reyes AA, Sjoquist MC, Magnotti L, Joseph B. Resuscitating the endothelial glycocalyx in trauma and hemorrhagic shock. Annals of Surgery Open. 2023;**4**(3):e298

[39] Wang G, Zhang H, Liu D, Wang X. Resuscitation fluids as drugs: Targeting the endothelial glycocalyx. Chinese Medical Journal. 2022;**135**(2):137-144

[40] Amgalan A, Allen T, Othman M, Ahmadzia HK. Systematic review of viscoelastic testing (TEG/ROTEM) in obstetrics and recommendations from the women's SSC of the ISTH. Journal of Thrombosis and Haemostasis [Internet]. 2020;**18**(8):1813-1838. DOI: 10.1111/jth.14882

[41] Liew-Spilger AE, Sorg NR, Brenner TJ, Langford JH, Berquist M, Mark NM, et al. Viscoelastic hemostatic assays for postpartum hemorrhage. Journal of Clinical Medicine. 2021;**10**(17):1-22

[42] Helms J, Iba T, Connors JM, Gando S, Levi M, Meziani F, et al. How to manage coagulopathies in critically ill patients. Intensive Care Medicine [Internet]. 2023;**49**(3):273-290. DOI: 10.1007/s00134-023-06980-6

[43] Snegovskikh D, Walton Z, Souzdalnitski D. Point-of-care thromboelastometry in the management

of acute obstetric hemorrhage. Current Obstetrics and Gynecology Reports [Internet]. 2016;**5**(3):244-249. DOI: 10.1007/s13669-016-0172-0

[44] Vlaar APJ, Dionne JC, de Bruin S, Wijnberge M, Raasveld SJ, van Baarle FEHP, et al. Transfusion strategies in bleeding critically ill adults: A clinical practice guideline from the European society of intensive care medicine. Intensive Care Medicine [Internet]. 2021;**47**(12):1368-1392. DOI: 10.1007/s00134-021-06531-x

[45] Malbrain MLNG, Martin G, Ostermann M. Everything you need to know about deresuscitation. Intensive Care Medicine [Internet]. 2022;**48**(12):1781-1786. DOI: 10.1007/s00134-022-06761-7

[46] Chawla LS, Davison DL, Brasha-Mitchell E, et al. Development and standardization of furosemide stress test to predict the severity of acute kidney injury. Critical Care. 2013;**17**:R207

[47] Chipman AM, Jenne C, Wu F, Kozar RA. Contemporary resuscitation of hemorrhagic shock: What will the future hold? Review article. American Journal of Surgery. 2020;**220**(January):580-588

[48] Zeng KW, Ovenell KJ, Alholm Z, Foley MR. Postpartum hemorrhage management and blood component therapy. Obstetrics and Gynecology Clinics of North America [Internet]. 2022;**49**(3):397-421. DOI: 10.1016/j.ogc.2022.02.001

[49] Carvajal JA, Ramos I, Kusanovic JP, Escobar MF. Damage-control resuscitation in obstetrics. The Journal of Maternal-Fetal & Neonatal Medicine. 2022;**35**(4):785-798. DOI: 10.1080/14767058.2020.1730800. Epub 2020 Feb 26

[50] Semple JW, Rebetz J, Kapur R. Transfusion-associated circulatory overload and transfusion-related acute lung injury. Blood. 2019;**133**(17):1840-1853

[51] Yu Y, Lian Z. Update on transfusion-related acute lung injury: An overview of its pathogenesis and management. Frontiers in Immunology. 2023;**14**:1175387

Chapter 3

Misoprostol, a Good Alternative for Preventing Postpartum Haemorrhage

De-Joseph Mibi Kakisingi

Abstract

Postpartum haemorrhage is the leading cause of maternal mortality. There are ways to prevent it and reduce the risk of maternal mortality. Oxytocin is the drug of first choice recommended by the WHO but poses problems in its conservation and management. Increasingly, misoprostol is recommended in place of oxytocin given the similar and sometimes superior results; it offers in preventing PPH and the ease of storage, transport, and ease of use that it offers. It offers comparison to oxytocin. Several studies have shown the effectiveness of misoprostol and its acceptance by both patients and medical staff.

Keywords: misoprostol, delivery, oxytocin, uterotonic, childbirth, postpartum haemorrhage, third stage of labor, active management of third stage, oxytocic drugs

1. Introduction

Maternal mortality is a global public health problem, with approximately 830 women dying every day worldwide from complications related to pregnancy or childbirth [1]. The maternal mortality ratio in developing countries in 2015 was 239 per 100,000 births, compared to 12 per 100,000 in developed countries [2].

Postpartum haemorrhage (PPH) is one of the leading causes of maternal death in sub-Saharan Africa. In developing countries, postpartum haemorrhage is responsible for 30% of maternal deaths [3].

Despite the identification of risk factors, postpartum haemorrhage (PPH) is most often unpredictable. The main causes of postpartum haemorrhage are uterine atony, placental insertion anomalies, and coagulation disorders [4].

Risk factors include multiple pregnancies, fetal macrosomia, primigravida, grand multiparity, older age, preterm births, genital tract injuries, non-use of uterotonic for PPH prophylaxis, labor induction, cesarean delivery, and intrauterine fetal deaths a history of postpartum haemorrhage. Uterotonics are used both for the prevention and treatment of postpartum haemorrhage if the cause is obviously uterine atony. Since then, several uterotonics have been proposed, some being more effective than others. Among the uterotonics, some require more complex and rigorous storage conditions. The routes of administration are also different for most of them. The WHO standard is "All women should benefit from the administration of a uterotonic at delivery to prevent delivery haemorrhage" [5, 6].

2. Anatomical reminders

The pregnant uterus at term consists of three muscular layers of unequal values. Due to pregnancy changes, the myometrium loses its complexity and approaches the embryonic and tubal structure. The superficial layer is specific to the uterine body. It is thin, subperitoneal, formed by longitudinal bundles in the midline and oblique laterally. The deep layer is made up of two sub-layers which are sandwiched in an intermediate zone. During pregnancy, this intermediate zone is covered by a rich venous plexus and muscular bundles whose predominant direction is transverse. Furthermore, these muscle bundles adhere to and surround the vessels. Thus, during contraction of the uterus the lumen of the vessels is erased. This device reduces haemorrhage to relatively small proportions of normal delivery.

Regarding vascularization, the uterine artery stretches, unwinds its turns, and increases its length, which triples or even quadruples. It is after delivery that the retraction of the uterine artery causes an increase in its caliber. It must be remembered that the flow rate of each uterine artery reaches 300 ml/min at the end of pregnancy (**Figure 1**) [7].

3. Physiological reminder

3.1 Physiology of the third phase of childbirth

Deliverance is the expulsion of the placenta and membranes from the genital tract. It progresses in three phases: placental abruption, expulsion of the placenta, and hemostasis.

Placental abruption phase: Placental abruption is dependent on uterine retraction which prepares it and uterine contractions which provoke it. Uterine retraction is a passive phenomenon, corresponding to the reduction in uterine volume during fetal expulsion. It results in an increase in thickness of the uterine walls respecting the area opposite the placental insertion which remains thin. This results in a physiological intermingling of the placenta, essential for its separation. Uterine

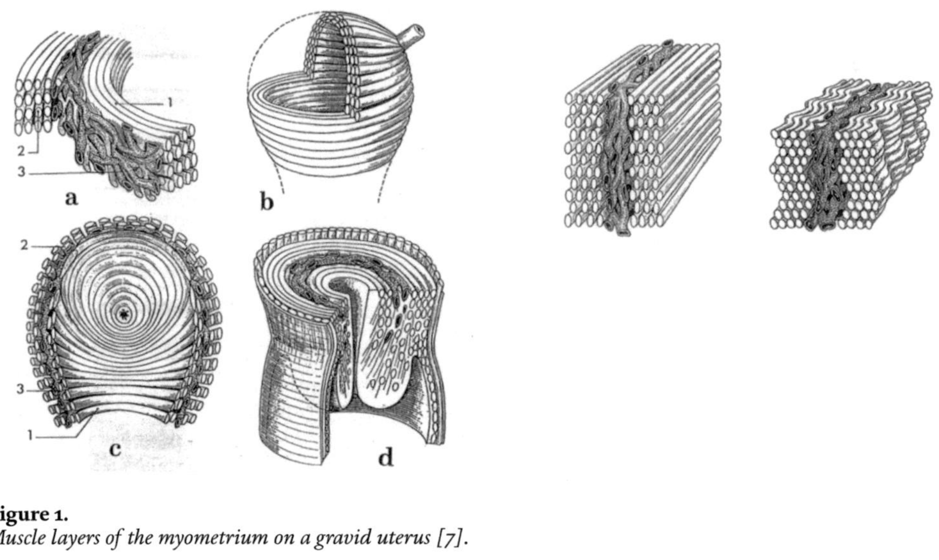

Figure 1.
Muscle layers of the myometrium on a gravid uterus [7].

contractions gradually increase in intensity. The physiologically enchatonated placenta, the perimeter of which is surrounded by a thicker muscular ring, undergoes concentric pressures which tend to make it bulge toward the cavity Uterine. This creates detachments in places, which will quickly lead to a retro-placental hematoma. Retroplacental hematoma results in complete cleavage between the uterine decidua (Superficial layer of the gravid uterine mucosa) and the deep mucosa layer which, remaining undamaged, will be the basis for the subsequent regeneration of the uterine mucosa.

Phase of migration and expulsion of the placenta: Under the influence of uterine contractions and its own weight, increased by the blood retained by the membranes still adhering to the uterine walls, the placenta falls into the lower segment which unfolds, lifting the uterine body. Then, the detached placenta then migrates through the cervix toward the vagina to be expelled to the vulva: Most frequently, through the fetal side of the placenta (BAUDELOCQUE mode), which occurs more often if the placenta is fundal or fairly high up; more rarely by its maternal side (DUNCAN mode), especially if it is low inserted. This method of delivery would promote complications (retained membranes, lower segment haemorrhage), requiring increased monitoring.

Uterine retraction phase: The phase of uterine retraction this time concerns the placental wound where it ensures hemostasis: the vessels are enclosed and closed by the contraction of the fibers Muscular; thrombosis occurring in these vessels is facilitated by coagulation factors, which are increased in late pregnancy. Blood loss is often underestimated.

3.2 Physiological hemostasis

Three factors are involved in uterine hemostasis:

Muscle factor: This is the most important mechanism because it is a fundamental locking system to stop bleeding. Hemostasis is essentially ensured by uterine retraction. The very strong retraction of the uterus closes the uterine vessels as they pass through the myometrium, closing the mesh of the plexiform layer. All the utero-placental vessels which until then nourished the placenta bleed but by contracting, the uterus tightens these vessels, and the bleeding ends up decreasing. At the area of insertion of the placenta in particular, the maternal vessels will find themselves enclosed and collapsing by the active contraction of the fibers of the myometrium which create a true physiological tourniquet or "living Pinard ligature". This is physiological vascular ligation of Pinard. Compression of the spiral arteries therefore limits intrauterine haemorrhage while compression of the venous sinuses will prevent the intrusion of amniotic fluid, tissue debris, air, and thromboplastinic substances into the maternal circulation. This uterine retraction will only be possible after complete evacuation of the uterus. It is this mechanism, and not the coagulation process, which is responsible for the rapid cessation of bleeding, so much so that, if the hemorrhagic risk is significant, it is useful to amplify this mechanism using utero tonics to reduce blood loss less than 150 ml ("directed" or "assisted" delivery).

Vascular factors: Prostaglandins, released by the endometrium after placental abruption, cause vasoconstriction. This reflex vasoconstriction reduces both the caliber and the flow.

Hemostatic factor: This factor can only work if the other two (2) are present. Thrombosis occurring in these vessels is facilitated by coagulation factors (fibrinogen, factors VII, VIII, and X) which are increased at the end of pregnancy.

3.3 Hormones and hemostasis

The essential phenomenon which explains physiological hemostasis is the contraction of the uterine muscles which occurs after childbirth. This contraction is induced by the action of certain hormones both to induce labor and to control the rhythm of uterine contractions and after expulsion, to ensure hemostasis by compressing the vessels that remain open. Two hormones play an important role in this phenomenon. These are oxytocin and prostaglandin. Oxytocin is a peptide hormone best known for its role in childbirth and breastfeeding. It is released in large quantities by the pituitary gland during labor and causes contractions of the uterus to facilitate birth. It also stimulates contractions during the third stage of labor: the separation of the placenta from the uterine wall and the compression of the maternal blood vessels after placental expulsion. When uterine contractions are not strong enough to compress the blood vessels, postpartum haemorrhage can threaten a woman's life. In this case, a woman will receive a utero tonic medication, to stimulate contractions and stop bleeding. Prostaglandins have recently appeared in the therapeutic armamentarium as an alternative to the surgical technique of hemostasis hysterectomy. Many authors have shown that plasma levels of endogenous prostaglandins reach a maximum at the time of delivery, 5–10 min after birth, and thus play a crucial role in uterine retraction [7]. The action of prostaglandins is more powerful and earlier than that of methylergometrine and oxytocin on the myometrium. Currently the mechanisms of action by which prostaglandins cause physiological hemostasis are known. Three types of prostaglandins are concerned: prostaglandins E2 and F 2 Alpha. These 2 types of prostaglandin are synthesized at the level of the amniochoreal membrane and the decidua. It crosses the placental barrier to trigger uterine contractions. Prostaglandin I 2 or prostacyclin is synthesized in the myometrium, and its role is to regulate uterine contractions. The uterine contractions induced by these two groups of prostaglandins will contribute to the regularity of labor and after the expulsion of the fetus and its appendages, to the reduction of haemorrhage by causing the uterine contractions which are at the origin physiological hemostasis by compression of the vessels.

4. Prevention of delivery haemorrhages

Preventing postpartum haemorrhage remains an absolute priority in obstetrics. Prevention of PPH is essential outside of a maternity ward as well as in the delivery room. Physiological means as described above are not enough to guarantee effective hemostasis and avoid haemorrhage which is the leading cause of maternal mortality despite prevention and treatment. Among postpartum haemorrhages (PPH), those during delivery are the most dangerous. This fear is reinforced by the fact that they represent the leading cause of maternal mortality and that their preventable nature reaches 50–80%, hence the importance of prevention by means that are effective and easy to handle. However, it should be noted that a haemorrhage of 500–1,000 ml is generally well tolerated with a clinical impact often only apparent beyond 1,000 ml of blood loss [7]. The prevention and even the management of haemorrhages during delivery use the means which make it possible to amplify the phenomenon of uterine contraction to achieve ligation of the uterine vessels by the plexiform muscles. For this purpose, utero tonics are used.

5. A toned uterus

(An oxytocic) is a product/medication that increases the tone of the muscles of the uterus. It stimulates the contraction of the uterine muscles. Drugs such as oxytocin and ergometrine have important uterotonic properties and have been used to treat uterine atony since their discovery. Oxytocin is the first-line medication for the management of postpartum haemorrhage. But more and more, misoprostol is used with results highly appreciated by many researchers.

5.1 Oxytocin and prevention of postpartum haemorrhage

SYNTOCINON® is a synthetic analogue of natural post-pituitary oxytocin. Oxytocin—or called oxytocin—is a cyclic nonapeptide. Physiologically, this hormone is synthesized by the hypothalamus, which projects its neuronal extensions into the posterior pituitary gland. This is where ADH and oxytocin will be stored to be released into the bloodstream when needed. Throughout pregnancy, and especially in the third trimester, stretching of the uterus and cervix sends impulses through afferent fibers to the hypothalamus. The latter responds by synthesizing oxytocin and delivering it through the posterior pituitary gland. Furthermore, its secretion is increased by stimulation of the breast and is reduced by taking ethanol. Its half-life in plasma is 5–10 min, and it is degraded by an amniopeptidase or oxytocinase and is eliminated by the kidney. It is at the end of pregnancy where we see an increase in estrogen levels which, on the one hand, stimulates the synthesis of oxytocin receptor in myometrial cells, and on the other hand, antagonizes the influence of progesterone. This is how the effectiveness of oxytocin increases during gestation: the uterus becomes more and more sensitive to its presence, due to the multiplication of receptors on the surface of muscle cells. Thus, oxytocin has the effect of acting mainly on the uterine smooth muscle and the mammary glands, by inducing an increase in the intracellular calcium concentration by stimulation of phospholipase C [1]. On the smooth muscle fiber, by increasing the intracellular calcium concentration, oxytocin increases the strength and frequency of muscle contractions. Indeed, once the hypothalamus is involved, positive feedback from oxytocin induces an increase in its secretion, and therefore, uterine contractions intensify and send feedback to the hypothalamus, and so on. Its action is coupled with that of prostaglandins, the synthesis of which by the placenta is induced by the secretion of oxytocin itself. It is therefore essential to avoid interfering with their production, for example, by using anti-prostaglandin drugs such as ibuprofen, which can then inhibit the first period of labor [8, 9]. Marketed under the name SYNTOCINON®, its composition is 5 IU of oxytocin per 1 mL ampoule.

5.1.1 Use in obstetrics and constraint

All women should benefit from the administration of a uterotonic during delivery to prevent PPH, and the recommended uterotonic is oxytocin (10 IU IV/IM). However, oxytocin requires a number of conditions for its conservation. The temperature sensitivity of oxytocin in solution requires that the injectable product be supplied and stored under refrigerated (2–8°C) (it should never be frozen) or cool (<25°C) to minimize degradation of oxytocin and maintain quality. This condition involves heavy logistics and rigor in conservation. In developed countries, this is already a significant challenge. In many low-resource countries temperatures will exceed 25°C, and cold chain infrastructure may be lacking or unreliable [10]. In some developing countries, the manufacture of oxytocin is not regulated as in developed countries; in addition, it is not always stored under proper temperature control, leading to deterioration of effectiveness, especially when exposed to sunlight and high temperatures. Oxytocin exists in injectable form only and requires the use of sterile consumables such as syringes, infusions, kits, etc., for its administration. It also requires the availability of trained medical personnel and medical supervision during its administration. Pain during injection is another factor that must be taken into account for the comfort of the patient.

5.2 Prostaglandins

Prostaglandins, natural and intrinsic substances, are revolutionizing all modern therapy. Since their discovery in 1913, they have continued to arouse a certain scientific curiosity on the part of researchers. In 1930, two American gynecologists, Kurszrok and Lieb, discovered that uterine strips from hysterectomized patients contracted or relaxed when exposed to human sperm [1]. A few years later, in 1934, Goldblatt in England and Von Euler in Sweden reported that seminal fluid and reproductive glands stimulated smooth muscle contraction. Von Euler identified the active material as a fat-soluble acid, capable of contracting certain smooth muscles and lowering blood pressure. He named this acid prostaglandin, believing that this hormone was secreted by the prostate. Von Euler's discovery was logical: we now know that seminal fluid is rich in prostaglandins, of the order of mg per ml. Everywhere else, their concentration is of the order of ng per ml [7]. In 1957, Bergstrôm's team isolated PGEl and PGFla in crystalline form. In 1964, this same team synthesized PGE2 from arachidonic acid. Therefore, numerous studies are devoted to the physiological effects of prostaglandins and make it possible to clarify, thanks to a series of discoveries, their role in the cardiovascular, digestive, respiratory, genitourinary systems, and the endocrine and nervous systems.

In 1968, Karim artificially induced labor in a woman, using an IV infusion of PGE2. But it was in the field of reproduction that prostaglandins aroused the interest of researchers in the 1970s. Their oxytocic properties and their action on the maturation and dilation of the cervix therefore gave rise to great hopes concerning their application in evacuation of uterine contents, prevention of postpartum haemorrhage, the process of cervical ripening, and artificial induction of labor.

5.2.1 Mechanism of action of prostaglandins

- *Membrane action*

At the cellular level, the initial step in the response to endogenous or exogenous prostaglandins appears to be binding to specific membrane receptors or to certain intracellular sites. The action of prostaglandins is essentially membrane-based, with the basis of controlling the activity of adenyl cyclase and/or guanyl cyclase, to form cAMP at the origin of the biological response from ATP or GTP. Other membrane enzymes (ATP-ases in particular) see their activity modulated by prostaglandins which thus intervene on membrane permeability to Ca^{2+} ions, hence the generation and propagation of action potentials at the origin of muscle contraction (**Figure 2**) [9].

- *Calcium and contractile system*

The myometrial response consists of an increase in the frequency of phasic contractile responses and an increase in baseline tone. Phasic contractions depend on the transmembrane influx of Ca^{2+} ions associated with brush action potentials:

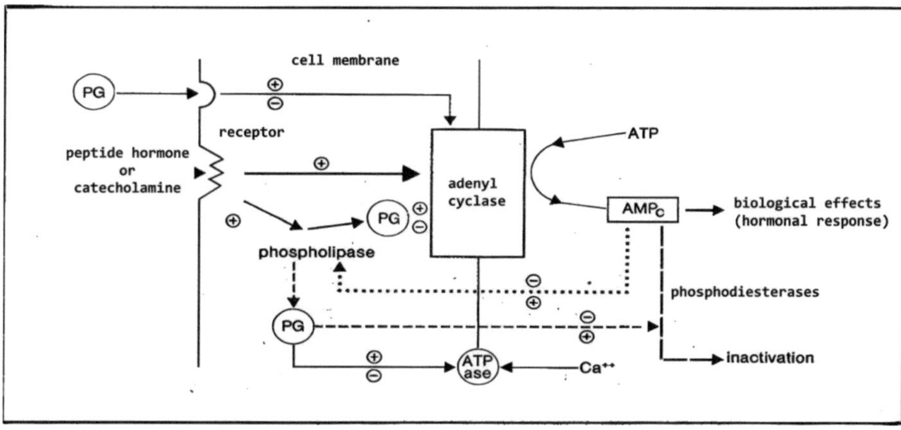

Figure 2.
Cellular mechanism of action of prostaglandins [9].

the ascending phase of the action potential is linked to the rapid entry of sodium and calcium. It is the concentration of intracellular calcium that regulates the contractile system. Calcium is essential for the establishment of uterine contraction, the sliding relative to each other of actin and myosin filaments requiring energy provided by hydrolysis of ATP. This hydrolysis is the result of a protein kinase having Ca^{2+} as a co-factor. Carsten demonstrated that for contractile proteins to be activated (by phosphorylation of a myosin light chain allowing the establishment of anchoring bridges between the myofilaments), the intracellular Ca^{2+} must be greater than 10-7 M [7].

On the other hand, the use of an inhibitor of an endoplasmic reticulum-dependent Ca^{2+}-ATPase, tBHQ (2,5-di(tert-butyl)-1,4-hydroquinone), led to a drop in the flux extracellular calcium and consequently a cessation of muscle contractions in vitro [8].

- *Messenger systems*

The cellular mechanism of action of prostaglandins at the level of myometrial cells can be explained by considering on the one hand the fundamental role attributed to calcium, but also on the other hand by highlighting the role of other messenger systems regulating contractile activity: – PGE2 and PGI2 stimulate adenyl cyclase and cAMP, – Phosphatidyl inositol (PI) promotes Ca^{2+} movements, di-acyl-glycerol (DAG) activates phospholipase A2, the importance of which is known for the synthesis of prostaglandins, and – Inositol tri phosphate (IP3), by mobilizing intracellular calcium, activates Ca^{2+}-Calmodulin-dependent protein kinases (Carsten) (**Figure 3**).

Messengers: IP3 and DAG, according to Tournaire.

Finally, we will note the contradiction manifested by prostaglandins E which cause both a contraction of the uterine fibers and an increase in intracellular cAMP. (cAMP causes the activation of a cAMP-dependent phosphorylase kinase involved in the inhibition of myosin light chain phosphorylation, promoting relaxation) (**Figure 4**).

Aucune source spécifiée dans le document actif [9].

5.2.2 Misoprostol and prevention of postpartum haemorrhage

Misoprostol is a medicine from the prostaglandin family. It is a synthetic prostaglandin, analogous to natural PGE1. Formerly used in the treatment of ulcers stomach

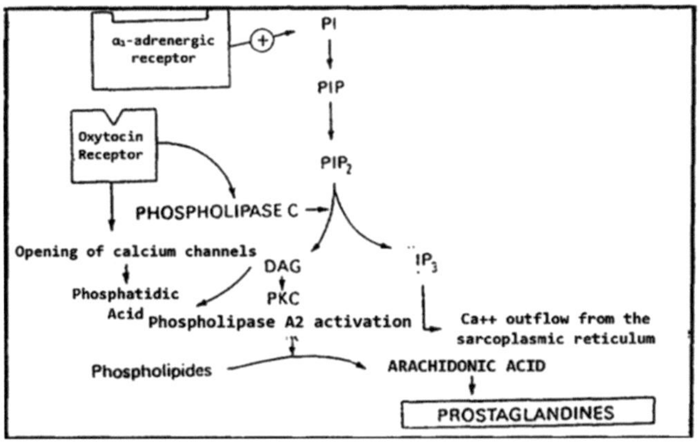

Figure 3.
Phosphatidyl inositol pathway with the second two [9]. PI, phosphatidyl inositol; PIP, phosphatidyl inositol 4-phosphate; PIP2, phosphatidyl inositol 4-5-phosphate; PKC, protein kinase C; IP3, inositol triphosphate; DAG, diacylglycerol; DAG, diacylglycerol.

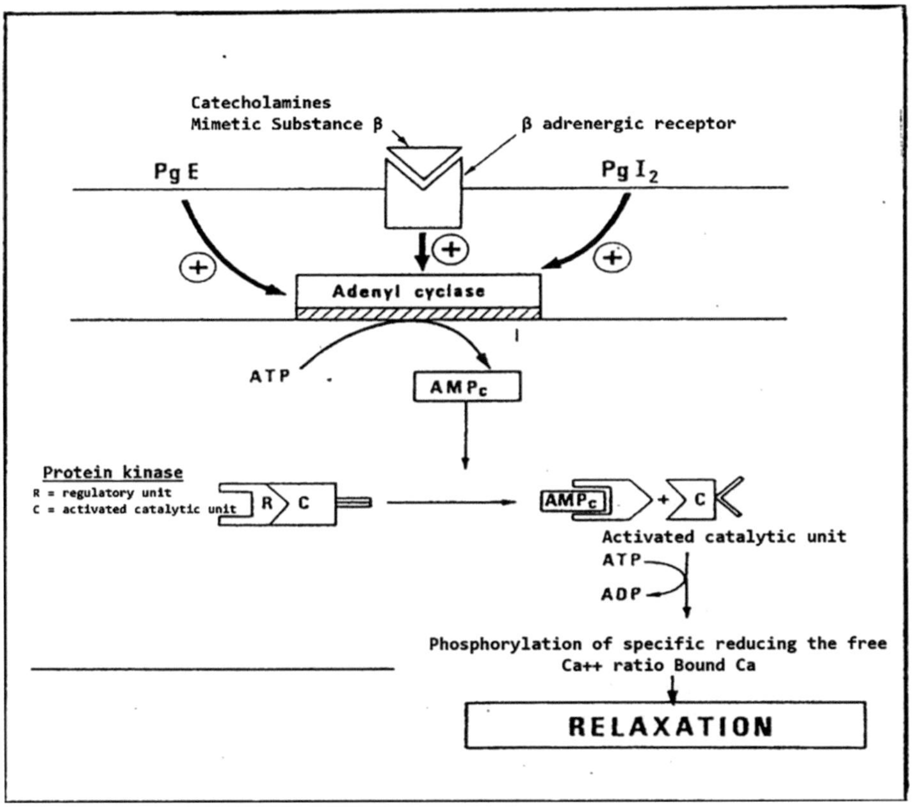

Figure 4.
Mode of action of certain myocontracting or muscle-relaxing substances whose final point of impact is the cAMP system, according to Tournaire. Cliquez ou appuyez ici pour entrer du texte. Aucune source spécifiée dans le document actif [9].

and duodenum and to prevent or treat gastritis due to non-steroidal anti-inflammatory treatment (NSAIDs). Today he has a double marketing authorization(AMM) for its use also in gynecology and obstetrics.

- *Therapeutic action*

In gynecology, at recommended doses, misoprostol causes contractions of the smooth muscle fibers of the myometrium and relaxation of the cervix. The uterotonic properties of misoprostol should facilitate the opening of the cervix and the expulsion of intrauterine debris. Through this mechanism, it allows hemostasis to be achieved also after childbirth. At recommended doses, misoprostol is not expected to cause cardiac, hepatic, or renal adverse effects. Misoprostol comes in tablets of 25 and 200 μg. Its use in gynecology and obstetrics is very broad. It is used both in the termination of pregnancy, the induction of labor, and in the prevention and treatment of postpartum haemorrhage. In the prevention of postpartum haemorrhage, doses of 200, 400, and 600 μg have been used according to the authors and research reaching similar conclusions but with different dose-dependent effectiveness. Studies using 600 μg had greater effectiveness in preventing postpartum haemorrhage. In the treatment of postpartum haemorrhage, FIGO recommends a dose of 800 μg.

- *Use in obstetrics and advantages*

Although the World Health Organization recommends the use of oxytocin for the prevention of PPH, the use of misoprostol is becoming more common due to its benefits in the management and treatment administration. Misoprostol, presented in tablet form, is indeed very easy to manage compared to oxytocin. Misoprostol does not need a cold chain, and it can be kept at room temperature below 25°C, which makes it easy to store and transport. Misoprostol can be stored for longer. It also offers several routes of administration. Misoprostol can be administered sublingually, rectally, and vaginally. Its administration does not require the presence of highly qualified personnel. At recommended doses, it has few side effects. For the treatment of postpartum haemorrhage, the rectal route is used when the sublingual route is impossible. A theoretical advantage of sublingual misoprostol could be better bioavailability achieved by avoiding first-pass metabolism [11]. Misoprostol appears to be a good alternative, but there is insufficient data on the comparative effectiveness of oxytocin 10 IU IM and sublingual misoprostol, particularly at the recommended dose of 600 mcg, for the prevention of PPH during active labor management.

6. Misoprostol, an evidence-based alternative

Oxytocin is rightly considered a first-line drug in the management of postpartum haemorrhage. This is because of the results obtained from its use and the fact that it is the most used medication throughout the world to prevent or treat postpartum haemorrhage. Misoprostol has been offered for several years as an alternative, especially in low-resource countries. Some practitioners remain skeptical, and scientists cite the absence of sufficient data to conclude. Since then, several studies have been conducted on the effectiveness of misoprostol in the prevention and management of postpartum haemorrhage. To be an alternative, misoprostol must provide at least the same level of effectiveness as oxytocin to be ethically accepted. Several studies were then carried out to verify this. The studies whose results are presented in this chapter consisted of comparing the effectiveness of misoprostol versus oxytocin in the prevention of postpartum haemorrhage. The samples included two groups. One group consisted of women given oxytocin treatment to prevent postpartum haemorrhage, and the other consisted of women given misoprostol treatment for the same cause. A study conducted on a sample of 652 cases, by Ballad et al., found that sublingual misoprostol was more effective than intramuscular oxytocin in reducing PPH [9]. A systematic review analysis carried out in Taiwan by Zümrüt Bilgin and Nuran Komürcü in 2019 that included 12 randomized controlled articles (n = 6290) concluded that in the misoprostol group, the rate of blood loss >500 mL was lower than that in the oxytocin group ($p < 0.05$). Misoprostol was found to be more effective than oxytocin in 10 out of 12 studies [12]. Another study conducted in India between 2012 and 2014, although on a small sample, noted a higher number of haemorrhages in the oxytocin group than in the misoprostol group [13]. A study conducted in the Democratic Republic of Congo, comparing misoprostol 600 μg sublingual to 10 IU of oxytocin IM in the prevention of postpartum haemorrhage, showed similar results. The study found that the proportion of PPH was higher in the group of women who received oxytocin 6.96% versus 2.87% in the group of women who received misoprostol (measured blood loss greater than 500 ml at 2 h).

After adjustment of this logistic regression model, a high probability of the occurrence of postpartum haemorrhages was noted in the groups of women who received oxytocin with a risk multiplied by 2.51 times that in the group of women having received misoprostol with a statistically significant difference ($p < 0.001$) [14]. Some studies have found that misoprostol is clinically equivalent to oxytocin when used to stop excessive postpartum bleeding suspected of being due to uterine atony in women who received oxytocin prophylactically at during the third phase of labor. A study done in Uganda in 2014 found a modest benefit from oxytocin compared to misoprostol. The Ugandan study found no significant differences in the rate of severe PPH, need for blood transfusion, postpartum hemoglobin, hemoglobin change, or use of supplemental uterotonics between the groups. study. The same study concludes that "the significant results between treatment groups also offer promising preliminary data that sublingual misoprostol at a dose of 600 mg is likely to be of significant benefit where oxytocin is not available".

These studies found that sublingual misoprostol was more effective than intramuscular oxytocin in reducing PPH [15–17]. The sublingual mode and/or powder formulation may increase the effectiveness of misoprostol and make it superior to injectable oxytocin for the prevention of PPH.

Other studies with a different objective to these have been carried out in certain areas of Asia and Africa. Among these studies, some have studied the practicality of misoprostol use by midwives who attend home births. Others have studied the possibility of distributing it to pregnant women living in remote areas, who do not have access to health facilities and who most often give birth in their homes. These are critical situations which unfortunately still exist in certain corners of the world. In a study carried out in the North-East department of Haiti, on "access to misoprostol for the prevention of postpartum haemorrhage at the level of health institutions and at home, the results clearly showed that the distribution community-based misoprostol is generally accepted by all stakeholders from the two municipalities. The satisfaction expressed by users of this product was also observed at all levels, whether providers, health workers, or community leaders. More than three quarters of women, or 79.2%, used misoprostol correctly after childbirth. The results revealed that the majority of women who received misoprostol in ANC and who delivered at home used it correctly" (USAID).

Misoprostol is easier to distribute among the local population than a less stable injectable medicine, such as oxytocin, to prevent or treat severe bleeding in women after childbirth (postpartum haemorrhage).

7. Conclusion

Misoprostol is a good alternative to oxytocin and offers more benefit in management, use, and distribution. For the prevention of PPH, a single dose of 600 μg (3 tablets of 200 μg) sublingual may be indicated, after the birth of the child, for the treatment of PPH secondary to uterine atony.

Author details

De-Joseph Mibi Kakisingi[1,2]

1 Evangelical University in Africa (UEA), Bukavu, Democratic Republic of the Congo

2 Saint Vincent Hospital Center, Bukavu, Democratic Republic of the Congo

*Address all correspondence to: dejokakis@gmail.com

References

[1] Alkema L, Chou D, Hogan D, Zhang S, Moller AB, Gemmill A, et al. Global, regional, and national levels and trends in maternal mortality between 1990 and 2015, with scenario-based projections to 2030: A systematic analysis by the UN maternal mortality estimation inter-agency group. Lancet. 2016;**387**:462-474. DOI: 10.1016/S0140-6736(15)00838-7

[2] Jacquot JM, Pouderoux P, Piat C, Strubel D. Prise en charge. Press Medicale. 2001;**30**:1645-1656

[3] Bagou G. Hémorragie du post-partum immédiat. Paris, France; 2012. Available from: https://www.sfmu.org/upload/70_formation/02_eformation/02_congres/Urgences/urgences2012/donnees/articles_titre/fs_conf21_art02.htm

[4] Muñoz M, Stensballe J, Ducloy-Bouthors AS, Bonnet MP, De Robertis E, Fornet I, et al. Patient blood management in obstetrics: Prevention and treatment of postpartum haemorrhage. A NATA consensus statement. Blood Transfus. Mar 2019;**17**(2):112-136. DOI: 10.2450/2019.0245-18. Epub 2019 Feb 6. PMID: 30865585; PMCID: PMC6476742

[5] OMS. Recommandations de l'OMS pour la prévention et le traitement de l'hémorragie du post-partum. 2014. 41 p. Available from: https://www.who.int/fr/publications-detail/9789241548502

[6] WHO Recommendations for the prevention and treatment of post-partum haemorrhage. 2014. 41 p. Available from: https://www.who.int/fr/publications-detail/9789241548502

[7] Kamina P. Anatomie gynécologique et obstétricale. Paris: Maloine s.a. editeur; 1979

[8] Atukunda EC, Siedner MJ, Obua C, Mugyenyi GR, Twagirumukiza M, Agaba AG. Sublingual misoprostol versus intramuscular oxytocin for prevention of postpartum hemorrhage in Uganda: A double-blind randomized non-inferiority trial. PLOS Medicine. 2014;**11**:e1001752. DOI: 10.1371/journal.pmed.1001752

[9] Hoarau M. Les prostaglandines en gynécologie-obstétrique: de l'interrruption de grossesse au déclenchement artificiel du tavail. Sciences Pharmaceutiques. 1997. 115 p. ffdumas-01344302f

[10] Lambert P, Nguyen TH, McEvoy C, Minhas RS, Wright P, Deadman K, et al. Quality of oxytocin ampoules available in health care facilities in the Democratic Republic of Congo: An exploratory study in five provinces. Journal of Global Health. 2018;**8**:020415. DOI: 10.7189/jogh.08.020415

[11] Aziz S, Kazi S, Haq G, Soomro N. Oral misoprostol versus oxytocin in the management of third stage of labour. The Journal of the Pakistan Medical Association. 2014;**64**:428-432

[12] Rani PR, Begum J. Recent advances in the management of major postpartum haemorrhage—A review. Journal of Clinical and Diagnostic Research. 2017;**11**:1-5. DOI: 10.7860/JCDR/2017/22659.9463

[13] Bellad M, Tara D, Ganachari M, Mallapur M, Goudar S, Kodkany B, et al. Prevention of postpartum haemorrhage with sublingual misoprostol or oxytocin: A double-blind randomised controlled trial. BJOG: An International Journal of Obstetrics and Gynaecology. 2012;**119**:975-986. DOI: 10.1111/j.1471-0528.2012.03341.x

[14] Mibi DJK, Nyakio O, Mbaya ÉI, Kakusu D, Musese MCN, Botalatala JB, et al. Comparative study of the efficacy of misoprostol and oxytocin Im in the prevention of post-partum haemorrhage in a low-resource setting. Open Journal of Obstetrics and Gynecology. 2023;**13**:983-996. DOI: 10.4236/ojog.2023.135083

[15] Priya GP, Veena P, Chaturvedula L, Subitha L. A randomized controlled trial of sublingual misoprostol and intramuscular oxytocin for prevention of postpartum hemorrhage. Archives of Gynecology and Obstetrics. 2015;**292**:1231-1237. DOI: 10.1007/s00404-015-3763-5

[16] Gallos ID, Papadopoulou A, Man R, Athanasopoulos N, Tobias A, Price MJ, et al. Uterotonic agents for preventing postpartum haemorrhage: A network meta-analysis. Cochrane Database of Systematic Reviews. 2018;**12**:CD011689. DOI: 10.1002/14651858.CD011689.pub3

[17] Mousa HA, Blum J, Abou El Senoun G, Shakur H, Alfirevic Z. Treatment for primary postpartum haemorrhage. Cochrane Database of Systematic Reviews. 2014;**9**:CD003249. DOI: 10.1002/14651858.CD003249.pub3

Chapter 4

Updates in Acute Respiratory Distress Syndrome

Dhaval Patel, Moyan Sun, Sandus Khan, Schaza Javed Rana and Andrew Strike

Abstract

Acute respiratory distress syndrome (ARDS) is a clinical entity characterized by widespread pulmonary injury following an inciting event. ARDS was first recognized in medical literature during the 1960s, and our knowledge of the disease and treatment has since then considerably advanced. The majority of patients who are diagnosed with ARDS ultimately require mechanical ventilation, and an estimated 10–15% of patients admitted to the intensive care unit (ICU) meet diagnostic criteria for severe ARDS. In this chapter, we present a comprehensive overview of ARDS with emphasis on the definition, etiology, pathophysiology, phenotypes, and management. The impact of medical innovations and scientific advances on the evolving definition of ARDS is explored through discussion of the parallels between medicine and technology. This concept is then linked to the myriad of ARDS etiologies which share a similar pathophysiological foundation. Expanding on this idea, we will focus on the ever-changing management of ARDS; importantly, this chapter will scrutinize the various viewpoints regarding mechanical ventilation strategies, prone ventilation, neuromuscular blockade, and extracorporeal membrane oxygenation (ECMO). This chapter concludes by discussion of prognosis and use of artificial intelligence in prognostication.

Keywords: acute respiratory distress syndrome (ARDS), acute hypoxemic respiratory failure, intensive care unit (ICU), mechanical ventilation, fluid therapies, neuromuscular blockade agents (NMBAs), extracorporeal membrane oxygenation (ECMO), prone ventilation, prognosis, practice guidelines

1. Introduction

ARDS is a clinical syndrome that is characterized by acutely worsening hypoxia with bilateral pulmonary infiltrates present on chest imaging after an inciting pulmonary injury [1, 2]. The COVID-19 pandemic has led to increased awareness and focus on ARDS due to the significant number of associated fatalities [2]. It is paramount to maintain a high index of clinical suspicion for ARDS in patients presenting with dyspnea, worsening hypoxemia, and characteristic findings on chest imaging to ensure prompt recognition and timely intervention. Unsurprisingly, up to 80% of patients who are diagnosed with ARDS will require mechanical ventilation, and an estimated 10–15% of patients will be admitted to the ICU, meeting diagnostic criteria for severe ARDS [1, 3]. In this chapter, we will be discussing etiology, pathophysiology, and management of ARDS. However, despite strides in diagnostic and therapeutic modalities on a global scale, ARDS remains a formidable, life-threatening disease process with an unwavering high mortality rate. Therefore, management guidelines are evolving as newer therapies are being explored.

2. Pathophysiology

2.1 Etiologies

The list of etiologies for ARDS is extensive and can be classified as infectious and non-infectious [1]. See **Table 1**. Sepsis is the most common infectious cause, while pancreatitis, aspiration of gastric contents, shock, and trauma are the most common non-infectious causes [1, 4]. There are several predisposing factors to ARDS such as smoking, alcohol, air pollution and genetics [5]. Genetic heterogeneity, although rare, may contribute towards sepsis. Haptoglobin variant Hp2 is an example of genetic association with risk of ARDS. This allele is predominant in 60% of people with European descent and thus subjecting them to an increased risk of ARDS [6].

2.2 Pathologic stages

ARDS develops through the activation of injury response pathways, involving inflammation and coagulation cascades, both locally in the lung and systemically [3, 4]. The hallmark pathological finding is diffuse alveolar damage caused by neutrophilic alveolitis and hyaline membrane deposition [5, 6]. The alveolar-capillary barrier is formed by Type I (AEC I) and Type II alveolar epithelial cells (AEC II) which intersperse one another. Injury to AEC I hinders fluid transport across the epithelium leading to alveolar flooding, while damage to AEC II type II impairs surfactant production [7, 8]. It is important to recognize that high tidal volumes and inspiratory pressures can further this injury by subjecting poorly compliant alveoli to volutrauma and barotrauma highlighting the importance of proper ventilator management in ARDS patients [9].

Pulmonary causes (direct lung injury)	Extrapulmonary causes (indirect lung injury)
• E-cigarettes, vaping	• Neurogenic
• Smoke inhalation	• Ischemic reperfusion after lung transplantation
• Drowning	• Pulmonary endarterectomy
• Aspiration	• Drug toxicity
• Pneumonia	• Transfusion-related acute lung injury
• Pulmonary Contusion	• Acute Pancreatitis
• Ventilator-induced lung injury	• Sepsis
	• Trauma
	• Fat/air embolism

Table 1.
Causes of acute respiratory distress syndrome [1].

Fluid-filled alveoli results in significant V/Q mismatch, inactivation of surfactant, and alveolar collapse [7, 8]. Subsequently, incomplete differentiation of AEC I from transitional cells leads to pulmonary fibrosis [10]. However, a recent study using explanted tissue from patients who underwent lung transplantation secondary to ARDS showed organized transitional cells (i.e., cuboidal, partially spread, flat cuboidal cells) without evidence of fibrosis. This suggests the possibility of clinical recovery and may justify the rationale of adequate treatment support including the use of extra-corporeal membrane oxygenation (ECMO), especially if patient is a candidate for lung transplant [11].

The pathogenesis of ARDS is thought to progress through three different stages: diffuse alveolar damage, proliferative stage, and finally, fibrotic stage. Diffuse alveolar damage usually happens in the first week of ARDS. By the time 2nd week of ARDS comes around, some degree of repair seems to start taking shape. In this proliferative stage, inflammation is resolved, neutrophils are removed, pulmonary edema is cleared, and alveolar-capillary membrane is restored.

However, when the inflammatory cascade persists, the myofibroblasts formed during the proliferative stage in the interstitium and responsible for deposition of extracellular proteins that help in repair, may lead to unabated fibrosis [12]. This process is like the process responsible for fibrotic damage in other organs, e.g., in kidneys [13].

2.3 Phenotyping

The process of grouping of ARDS into homogenous groups is called phenotyping and it aids in streamlining relevant treatment options [14]. Phenotypes can be further classified into sub phenotypes. This is a topic that needs considerable future research. Two sub phenotypes of biological and radiological origin are further described below.

Biologic phenotypes are further classified as hyper and hypo inflammatory. Hyperinflammatory sub-phenotypes have higher IL-6, IL-8, and TNF receptor-1 but lower bicarbonate and protein C concentration as compared to hypo inflammatory [15, 16]. Hyperinflammatory ARDS is associated with longer ICU stay, fewer ventilator-free days and higher 90- days mortality thus highlighting the importance of understanding the biological phenotypes in management [15, 16]. Radiologic phenotypes use the modality of computed tomography (CT) to further classify ARDS as diffuse and patchy loss of aeration vs. predominant dorsal-inferior consolidation. The former responds well to alveolar recruitment strategies while the latter has better outcome with proning [17]. A randomized control trial (RCT) showed personalized treatment based on radiologic phenotyping decreased mortality by 10% [18]. In future, phenotyping may allow for individually tailored treatment strategies and hopefully, better outcomes [19].

3. Diagnosis

Since its inception, the diagnostic criteria of ARDS have undergone many revisions. The 2012 Berlin definition, as noted in **Table 2**, played an essential role in providing feasible, reliable parameters that could objectively define ARDS. It improved the predictive validity for mortality compared to the previous definition by the American-European Consensus Conference (AECC) [20, 21]. The Berlin criteria improved specificity, established the severity of oxygenation, and acknowledged the

Timing	• Within 1 week of known clinical insult or new respiratory symptoms
Chest imaging	• Bilateral opacities not fully explained by effusions, lobar/lung collapse, or nodules (on chest x-ray or chest computed tomography)
Origin of edema	• Respiratory failure not fully explained by cardiac failure or fluid overload. • Requires objective assessment (e.g., TTE) to exclude cardiogenic pulmonary edema if no risk factors present
Oxygenation	• Mild: PaO_2/FiO_2 200-300 mmHg with PEEP or CPAP $\geq$5 cm H_2O • Moderate: PaO_2/FiO_2 101-199 mmHg with PEEP $\geq$5 cm H_2O • Severe: $PaO_2/FiO_2 \leq 100$ mmHg with PEEP $\geq$5 cm H_2O

Abbreviations: CPAP: continuous positive airway pressure; FiO_2: fraction of inspired oxygen; PaO_2: partial pressure of arterial oxygen; and PEEP: positive end-expiratory pressure.

Table 2.
Acute respiratory distress syndrome: Berlin criteria [20].

role of noninvasive ventilation (NIV) in mild ARDS. However, after global adoption, many limitations became clear—specifically, the exclusion of patients in locations where NIV or invasive ventilation is unavailable, the lack of noninvasive oximetry as equivalent to PaO_2 on arterial blood gas (ABG), and the lack of high-flow nasal oxygen (HFNO) incorporation [20–22]. The results of the FLORALI trial have shifted the paradigm in favor of NIV in hypoxemic respiratory failure [22]. There are other limitations to Berlin 2012 definition, such as use of chest radiographs, which have compared poorly to CT chest (SN 0.73, SP 0.70, PPV 0.88, NPV 0.47) [20, 22, 23]. Also, when Berlin criteria is matched with biopsies from patients, the criteria has low specificity for ARDS [21]. Finally, the mortality prediction is poor, but improved compared to AECC. Based on a meta-analysis of 4188 patients – Berlin ROC AUC = 0.577 compared to 0.536 for AECC [20]. The Kigali modification recognized these limitations and emerged to address practical constraints in resource-limited regions, yet it did not reach the global adoption seen by the Berlin definition [20, 21]. See **Figure 1**.

In 2023, the Matthay modification (**Figure 1**) aimed to rectify the known limitations of the Berlin definition. Notable modifications include an extended onset of

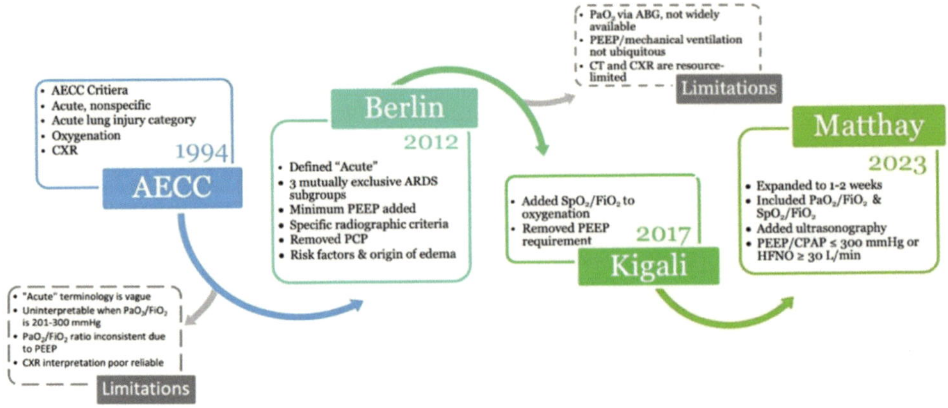

Figure 1.
Evolution and timeline of ARDS diagnostic criteria [21, 22].

opacities following the initial insult (1–2 weeks) to encompass more indolent diseases like COVID-19, incorporation of ultrasonography for detecting bilateral opacities addresses resource limitations in regions where CT imaging or chest X-rays may not be readily available, the use of SpO2/FiO2 as an alternative to the PaO2/FiO2 ratio, with the advantage of noninvasive pulse oximetry's widespread availability, and lastly, the inclusion of non-intubated patients on HFNO who meet ARDS criteria, requiring at least 30 L/min, expanding the criteria for invasive or noninvasive ventilation [21, 22].

4. Ventilation

4.1 Non-invasive ventilation

NIV includes simple face mask, nasal canula, non-rebreather, HFNO, continuous positive airway pressure (CPAP), bilevel positive airway pressure (BiPAP) and helmet ventilation. It is used in patients with mild ARDS who are hemodynamically stable or severe ARDS if patient can maintain oxygenation without the need for intubation. However, a large observational study, LUNG SAFE trial showed use of NIV in patients with severe ARDS was associated with higher ICU mortality [24]. Another prospective study on NIV use in ARDS showed slower recovery in patients with pulmonary ARDS vs. extrapulmonary cause [25].

4.2 Mechanical ventilation

Most patients with ARDS end up requiring mechanical ventilation. There are certain evidence-based ventilation practices that are recommended in ARDS. We will visit them next.

4.2.1 FiO2

During and after intubation, care must be taken to prevent hyperoxia to further prevent collapse of alveoli with low V/Q ratio [26]. Adverse effects of oxygen are dose and duration of exposure dependent. For e.g., in rat models mortality rapidly decreases once fio2 is lowered from 100 to 85% [27]. While Fio2 is set at 100% initially, in accordance with ARDSNet, recommendation is to maintain saturation (SpO2) of 88–95% which corelates with an arterial oxygen tension (PaO2) between 55 to 80 mmHg. The recommended goal is conservative oxygenation. No mortality benefit has been found in trials comparing conservative with liberal oxygen therapy targeting PaO2 90 to 105 mmHg: SpO2 $\geq$ 96% [28].

4.2.2 Low tidal volume ventilation

The gold standard approach of mechanical ventilation in ARDS has been laid down by the famous ARDSNet study (ARMA). It compared the use of standard tidal volume (Vt) of 12 mL/kg with low tidal volume ventilation (LTVV) between 4 and 8 mL/kg while aiming for a plateau pressure (P_{plat}) $\leq$ 30 cm of H2O. The weight in kg is predicted body weight. The study showed a decrease in ventilator-induced lung injury (VILI) and 22% reduction in mortality [29]. Despite the compelling evidence, LTVV is underutilized. A prospective cohort in 2016 showed only 60% clinicians successfully diagnosing ARDS and less than two thirds of those diagnosed received LTVV [1, 29]. One part of LTVV strategy is targeting high PEEP, and the other is keeping plateau pressure ≤ 30 mmHg.

4.2.3 PEEP

PEEP plays a key role in alveolar recruitment and oxygenation. As noted above, high PEEP is a part of LTVV. ALVEOLI and LOVS trials demonstrated the use of high PEEP. In ARMA trial, PEEP was high but set according to Fio2 [30, 31]. According to the ALVEOLI trial high PEEP improved oxygenation on Day 1 and Day 3 of admission but showed no difference in ventilator free days and mortality as compared to low PEEP. A meta-analysis showed mortality benefit when higher PEEP strategy was used without recruitment maneuver [32]. Another meta-analysis, a Cochrane review, showed reduced mortality in patients with moderate to severe ARDS but increased mortality in mild ARDS [33]. Based on these two meta-analyses, American Thoracic Society (ATS) made a conditional recommendation for the use of high PEEP without recruitment maneuvers in patients with moderate to severe ARDS [34].

There are many ways PEEP can be titrated such as using FiO2 as in ARMA trial, measuring esophageal pressures, looking at the inflection points on pressure-volume loops, using lung ultrasound or by calculating maximum oxygen delivery. No one measure has proven to be more beneficial than others. Optimal PEEP is still a matter of debate at this point. In general, it is recommended that initial PEEP be set at 5-8 cm of H_20 for hypoxic respiratory failure and a higher PEEP but not higher than 34 cm of H_20 for moderate to severe ARDS. The higher PEEP should be individualized based on patient's compliance, oxygenation status and hemodynamics.

4.2.4 Recruitment maneuvers

To maintain or maximize alveolar oxygenation, recruitment maneuvers may be used. It usually means applying a positive pressure such as 35–40 cm of H2o for an extended duration, e.g., 20–40 seconds. Optimal time to apply recruitment maneuvers is when patient has derecruited such as after transport. Another such maneuver is Sigh Ventilation which is a cyclic maneuver. For this strategy, enough tidal volume is applied to produce a sufficient plateau pressure such as 35 cm of H2O every few minutes. The SiVent Randomized Clinical Trial was undertaken to figure out whether adding sigh ventilation improved clinical outcomes in patients with trauma who were at risk for ARDS. Although the trial did not suggest any difference in ventilator free days, prespecified secondary outcomes suggested mortality benefit [35]. Recently, there were two trials that evaluated the use of high PEEP applied for prolonged duration as a recruitment maneuver in ARDS patients. One trial found it increased mortality, and another found that it increased rates of cardiac arrythmia, but neither found any benefit [36, 37]. Based on these trials, ATS recommended against the use of lung recruitment maneuvers in moderate to severe ARDS [34].

4.2.5 Modes of ventilation

The two common modes of ventilation are Volume (VC) vs. Pressure Control (PC). Evidence does not support one mode over another. The preference usually comes down to practice pattern. The goals are to minimize patient's work of breathing with the hope that will further prevent cascading inflammation and decrease the

DOI: http://dx.doi.org/10.5772/intechopen.1004721

ongoing acute lung injury, aim for LTVV, keep airway pressures (plateau and driving pressures) in check to prevent further ventilation induced lung injury and prevent hyperoxia as described above.

There is another mode, Auto Pressure Release Ventilation (APRV) that is sometimes used in practice. The concept of APRV revolves around a specific time switching mode alternating between long duration of high airway pressure (T high) and short duration of low airway pressure (T low). By using the biphasic Positive airway pressure (BIPAP), APRV may help reduce barotrauma by minimizing alternating recruitment and de-recruitment of alveoli. Other advantages may include increased functional residual capacity, unrestricted spontaneous breathing resulting in improved ventilation/perfusion(V/Q) mismatch and decreased need for sedation and neuromuscular blockade [38–40]. A single center randomized controlled trial by Zhou et al. showed superiority of APRV over LTVV in terms of improving oxygenation and compliance, decreasing plateau pressure, and reducing the duration of mechanical ventilation and ICU stay in patients with ARDS [41]. There is still a dearth of solid data in medical patients to recommend usage of APRV over LTVV. However, it may be a suitable ventilation strategy in selective patients and may be useful depending on the experience of the providers.

4.2.6 Respiratory rate

In addition to LTVV at 6 mL/kg, the initial respiratory rate (RR) is set at ≤35, adjusted to meet the demands of minute ventilation (commonly ranging between 14 and 22 breaths/minute) [29]. Respiratory rate is an integral part of mechanical power which is discussed below.

4.2.7 Driving pressure and mechanical power

Driving Pressure (DP) calculation is useful in patients with moderate to severe ARDS. DP is equal to ventilator measured P_{plat} minus applied positive end-expiratory pressure (PEEP) or Tidal volume (VT)/ respiratory system compliance. A retrospective analysis of nine trials including 3562 patients on mechanical ventilation for ARDS proved that DP was the best predictor of survival when compared to VT, PEEP and P_{plat}. A DP increase in 7 cm of H2O was associated with increased mortality [42]. Usually, a target DP of < or = 14 cm of H2O has shown clinical benefits [43].

Lately, a unifying concept has emerged-Mechanical Power (MP). In simple words, it is the collective energy delivered by the ventilator to the patient. Therefore, it can be hypothesized that lower MP may increase the odds for better outcomes.

The mechanical power in Volume and Pressure Controlled mode are described in the following equations (Eqs. (1) and (2)):

$$\mathrm{VC:MP} = \mathrm{RR}.\left\{\Delta V^2.\left[1/2.\mathrm{EL}_{rs} + \mathrm{RR}.(1+\mathrm{I:E})/60.\mathrm{I:E}.\mathrm{R}_{aw}\right] + \Delta V.\mathrm{PEEP}\right\} \quad (1)$$

where ΔV is the tidal volume, EL_{rs} is the elastance of the respiratory system, *I:E* is the inspiratory-to-expiratory time ratio, and R_{aw} is the airway resistance [44].

$$\mathrm{PC:MP} = 0.098^{*}\ \mathrm{RR}^{*}\ \mathrm{V}_t^{*}\left[\mathrm{PEEP} + \Delta \mathrm{P}_{insp}^{\ *}\left(1 - e^{*} - \mathrm{Tinsp}/\mathrm{R}^{*}\mathrm{C}\right)\right] \quad (2)$$

where 0.098 is a conversion factor to J/min, RR is the respiratory rate in beats/min, V_t is the tidal volume in L, PEEP is the positive-end expiratory pressure in cmH_2O, ΔP_{insp} is the inspiratory pressure in cmH_2O, T_{insp} is the inspiratory time in s, R is the resistance in $cmH_2O/L/s$ and C is the compliance in L/cmH_2O [45].

To figure out each ventilator variable's impact, 4549 patients from a pooled database were analyzed [26]. Results showed only two variables, DP, and RR, had a significant association with mortality. The effect of every 1 cm H2O increase in driving pressure produced 4 times the effect of increase in each breath/min of RR. This can be summed into a bivariate model represented by the equation: {(4*DP) + RR}; this was a significant predictor of mortality even more so than mechanical power and may hold the independent variables that truly predict mortality in the mechanical power equation [26].

Chiumello et al. derived simplified equations for both VC and PC that can be used for bedside calculation and found they had good correlation with the above-mentioned equations [46]. The equations are described below (Eqs. (3) and (4)).

$$VC: MP = \left\{ VE^{*} (\text{Peak Pressure} + \text{PEEP} + \text{Inspiratory flow} / 6) \right\} / 20 \quad (3)$$

where VE is the minute ventilation expressed in l/min. Peak pressure and PEEP are expressed in cmH_2O.

$$PC: MP = 0.098^{*} RR^{*} V_t^{*} \left[PEEP + \Delta P_{insp} \right] \quad (4)$$

where 0.098 is a conversion factor from $cmH_2O\ l\ min^{-1}$ in J/min, RR is the respiratory rate, and V_t is the tidal volume in liters. PEEP and ΔP_{insp} is the pressure (cmH_2O) above PEEP during pressure-controlled ventilation.

In a proof-of-concept study, Petra J et al., showed that VC without pause time had the lowest mechanical power [47]. Overall, mechanical power remains an exciting concept that may offer a unifying variable that can be targeted to decrease the risk of VILI. Further research will be needed to validate this concept for bedside use.

4.2.8 Side effects of mechanical ventilation

The four common pathophysiological mechanisms associated with VILI include atelectrauma, barotrauma, volutrauma and biotrauma [48]. Atelectrauma involves damage to the alveolar unit caused by high-shear forces that help in the recruitment of alveoli. Interalveolar septae and fluid-filled nonaerated alveoli mediate the deformation of neighboring alveolar units, resulting in trauma [48]. Barotrauma is caused by high lung inflation pressure, leading to regional overdistention of the alveolar unit resulting in alveolar rupture, pneumothorax, pneumomediastinum, and subcutaneous emphysema. Volutrauma results from alveolar over-distension. Biotrauma results from the release of cytokine and inflammatory mediators due to mechanical injury. This not only affects normal and diseased lungs, but may result in multi organ dysfunction [48, 49].

LTTV is associated with potential side effects including but not limited to hypercapnia, auto-PEEP, ventilator dyssynchrony and as previously described, VILI. Hypercapnic respiratory acidosis is the result of alveolar hypoventilation to avoid overdistention. Studies have shown that permissive hypercapnia may be beneficial when LTVV is applied [50].

Theoretically, LTVV needs a higher respiratory rate which may result in auto-PEEP due to insufficient time of expiration. Subgroup analysis from ARDSNet trial detected insignificant auto-PEEP (needs source). LTVV may result in increased work of breathing that may result in increased sedation requirement at the initiation of LTVV. The need for increased sedation does not usually persist [51].

A common phenomenon experienced in one quarter of mechanically ventilated patients is dyssynchrony described as incongruity between the patients' breathing efforts and ventilator- delivered breaths [52–54]. Factors affecting dyssynchrony can be divided into patient- centered and ventilator centered. Patient's factors include respiratory drive and lung mechanics (compliance and airflow resistance). Ventilator factors include respiratory rate, inspiratory flow, and trigger sensitivity. Double triggering (breath stacking) commonly seen in ARDS occurs when the second breath is taken before the ventilator completes the first breath [55]. Increasing the VT while maintaining the 4 to 8 mL/kg and recommended P_{plat} may help with the problem. Ineffective triggering results from a failed effort on patient's part to trigger the ventilator and may suggest presence of auto PEEP. Reverse triggering involves mechanical ventilation induced contractions. Decreasing sedation, increasing sedation, neuromuscular blockade or adjusting the respiratory rate or tidal volume may help alleviate some of the problems.

5. Fluids

Fluids are a common topic of discussion in ARDS, and in the past have often been the source of some controversy. Studies have shown that a conservative, rather than a more liberal approach, leads to more favorable outcomes [56, 57]. Given increased vascular permeability, a conservative approach to fluids is needed, with the goal of minimizing or eliminating a positive fluid balance, if patients are hemodynamically stable [57]. Although difficult to achieve in clinical practice, literature suggests aiming for a central venous pressure (CVP) of <4 mmHg or a pulmonary artery occlusion pressure (PAOP) of <8 mmHg [56]. Conservative fluid strategy, consisting of fluid restriction and use of diuretics, leads to improvement in oxygenation index, lung injury score and increased numbers of ventilator-free days and ICU-free days [57]. Although a clear mortality benefit has not been proven, retrospective data suggests a positive fluid balance is associated with increased 30-day mortality compared to a negative fluid balance [57, 58]. The high-inflammatory phenotype, which is associated with higher mortality, seems to benefit from conservative fluid strategy the most [58].

6. Prone ventilation

Prone ventilation is a technique in which ventilation is delivered while a patient is placed in a prone position. Prone position reduces the difference between dorsal and ventral transpulmonary pressure, recruits alveoli that collapse during supine ventilation and decreases medial posterior lung compression [59, 60]. These effects improve ventilation and oxygenation by increased lung recruitment [60]. Proning may also decrease systemic inflammation.

Current recommendations stemming from PROSEVA trial suggest that after a 12–24 hours of stabilization period with supine ventilation, prone ventilation can be initiated for up to 36 hours for patients with severe ARDS [61]. Per the PROSEVA trial, the mean duration of time in prone position was 17 hours per session with an average of 4 sessions. Most patients who show a response to prone positioning usually do so within the first hour after being placed into the prone position [61]. A response can be [determined] via improvement in ABG of >10 mmHg PaO2 on ventilator after 1 hour or notable increase in lung compliance based on a decrease in plateau pressure [62].

PROSEVA trial showed decrease in mortality in patients with severe ARDS who undergo prone ventilation [61]. It also showed improvements in ventilator-free days and time to extubation. Proning does not seem to prevent organ dysfunction or lead to reduced ICU stay [61, 62]. Several meta-analyses concur on the findings of PROSEVA trial, with one meta-analysis even reporting that proning of 12 hours or more in patients with severe ARDS led to lower mortality [63]. This suggests that at least 12-hours of proning session daily is sufficient to provide benefit of reducing mortality [63].

Contraindications and complications of proning are outlined below in **Table 3** [63]. Of note, use of prone positioning in an ICU is a labor-intensive process as staff need experience and training as they should be able to quickly put patient back into supine positioning, for e.g., to perform cardiopulmonary resuscitation [64].

In the light of COVID-19 pandemic, prone positioning in awake patients who are not intubated has garnered much attention. Recent data shows that prone positioning reduced the need for intubation for patients with COVID-19 induced acute hypoxemic respiratory failure and should be used in patients with COVID-19 that are in the ICU or are requiring advanced respiratory support [65]. Awake COVID-19 patients who are on supplemental oxygen but do not require mechanical ventilation may not have the same clinical benefits from prone positioning and have a high probability of worse clinical outcomes [65]. Therefore, prone positioning should not be used on all patients with COVID-19 but rather, be individualized based on degree of hypoxic respiratory failure. The considerations for initiation of the use of prone positioning, the length and its discontinuation in COVID-19 patients are like non-COVID-19 ARDS patients. However, prone positioning in awake patient does not have enough data to extrapolate to those with non-COVID ARDS and further trials are called for [66].

Absolute contraindications	Relative contraindications	Complications
• Spinal instability, including patients at risk of spinal instability (i.e., History of rheumatoid arthritis) • Unstable fractures • Anterior burns • Open wounds in places that would limit proning • Pregnancy • Acute bleeding	• Severe hemodynamic instability (i.e., on multiple pressors) such that patient is not able to tolerate change in positioning • Active arrythmias that may require cardioversion • Recent thoracic &/or abdominal surgeries	• Pressure injuries • Facial edema • Transient reduction in oxygen saturation • Transient arrhythmias

Table 3.
Contraindications and complications of prone ventilation [63].

Recently completed, PRONECMO trial concluded that prone ventilation did not significantly reduce time to successful weaning of ECMO for patients with severe ARDS supported by VV-ECMO when compared to supine position [67].

7. Steroids

The proposed indications glucocorticoid in ARDS varies among professional society guidelines. It is widely accepted that glucocorticoids, specifically dexamethasone, are likely to benefit patients with moderate to severe ARDS during the early course of disease. Before the DEXA-ARDS trial in 2020, many studies had demonstrated fewer ventilator days and shorter ICU length of stay with steroid use [68]. This was further supported by the DEXA-ARDS trial in 2020 which once again showed that in patients with moderate to severe ARDS as defined by PaO_2/FiO_2 of 100–200, early dexamethasone usage improved ventilatory-free days and decreased mortality [68]. The intervention of DEXA-ARDS, which dictates most of current practice, was dexamethasone 20 mg IV daily for days 1–5, followed by 10 mg daily from days 6–10; following extubation, dexamethasone was stopped [68]. It should be noted that steroids should not be used in Influenza related ARDS as it is associated with higher mortality [69].

8. Neuromuscular blockade

The mitigating effects of neuromuscular blockade agents (NMBAs) on inflammation, oxygen consumption, and ventilatory dyssynchrony intrinsic to the pathophysiology of ARDS have long been theorized. However, earlier research has not substantiated this hypothesis. Despite its arguable potential, the widespread adoption of NMBAs among ICUs is still limited, presenting an intriguing avenue for further investigation.

The first multicenter trial was ACURASYS 2010 [70]. It showed that in patients with severe ARDS (i.e., PaO2/FiO2 ≤ 120 mmHg), the use of cisatracurium improved adjusted 90-day mortality and increased ventilatory-free days. However, no statistically significant difference was seen in crude 90-day, 28-day, in-hospital, or ICU mortality rates. Furthermore, whether cisatracurium or heavy sedation caused these differences could not be concluded as all patients were heavily sedated.

The second multicenter trial was ROSE in m019 [71]. See **Table 4**. It randomized patients with moderate to severe ARDS (i.e., PaO2/FiO2 ≤ 150 mmHg) with PEEP of ≥8 cm H2O to receive cisatracurium vs. placebo randomly, but the trial stopped early after enrolling 1006 patients due to futility. ROSE 2019 concluded that compared to placebo, cisatracurium did not significantly reduce 90-day in-hospital mortality (42% cisatracurium vs. 43% control; P = 0.93). Furthermore,

	ROSE	ACURASYS
Prone ventilation	• 15.8%	• 44.8%
Sedation targets	• Light sedation	• Heavy sedation
PEEP strategies	• Higher	• Lower
Abbreviation: PEEP = positive end-expiratory pressure.		

Table 4.
Differences between ROSE and ACURASYS trials [70, 71].

secondary outcomes at day 28 (e.g., in-hospital mortality, ventilatory-free days, and ICU-free days) also showed no significant difference. Moreover, the cisatracurium group had significantly more complications of ICU-acquired weakness and serious adverse cardiovascular events [71]. ROSE not only cast doubt on the beneficial effects of early NMBAs for patients with moderate to severe ARDS but also suggested potential harm.

European Society of Intensive Care Medicine (ESICM) published its guidelines in 2023 and recommended against the routine use of NMBAs in moderate-t0-severe ARDS [72]. ESICM noted that given differing ventilatory approaches between the two trials and heavy use of sedation in ACURASYS, NMBA cannot be recommended in ARDS patients.

9. Extracorporeal membrane oxygenation (ECMO)

Despite the other evidence-based modalities mentioned in this chapter, severe ARDS is still associated with high mortality [73]. In the last decade, with the widespread adoption of ECMO around U.S., it has become an intervention that is often considered for patients with severe ARDS. However, lack of universal availability of ECMO and limited circuits of ECMO at ECMO centers has prevented ECMO from becoming a routine standard of care for patients with severe ARDS.

COVID-19 pandemic has accelerated the use of ECMO [74]. The goal of implementing ECMO in ICU care is to provide advanced mechanical life support to patients with acute respiratory or cardiac failure [75]. This support is achieved by draining deoxygenated blood from the venous system via cannulation, pumping the blood through a membrane that facilitates oxygen and carbon dioxide exchanges, and returning the newly oxygenated blood to the body for circulation and organ perfusion. The two most utilized ECMO cannulation strategies are venovenous (VV) and venoarterial (VA), which provide isolated respiratory support and combined cardiopulmonary support, respectively [75]. In the setting of ARDS, VV ECMO is the strategy that is commonly implemented. Because of this, the current landmark trials evaluating implementation of ECMO in ARDS have focused on VV cannulation (**Figures** 2 and **3**).

9.1 The ECMO trials

CESAR (Conventional Ventilation or ECMO for Severe Adult Respiratory Failure) trial showed a statistically significant improvement in survival rates by 33–35% without disability in the group evaluated for ECMO when compared to conventional ventilation [76]. The other trial, EOLIA (ECMO to Rescue Lung Injury in Severe ARDS) randomized patients to conventional ventilation or VVECMO in severe ARDS [77]. It showed no mortality benefit. However, multiple secondary outcomes did show significant improvement with the early ECMO intervention group. These outcomes included ICU length of stay, days free from mechanical ventilation, and days free from renal replacement therapy. In the intention-to-treat analysis, mortality at 60 days was 35% (44 out of 124) in the ECMO arm and 46% (57 out of 125) in the control arm; a relative risk of 0.76 (95% CI 0.55–1.04) with p-value of 0.09. This meant an absolute risk reduction of 11% in the ECMO arm, but this did not reach statistical significance [77]. A post hoc analysis of EOLIA trial showed mortality benefit, but the range of benefit varied depending on the analysis [78].

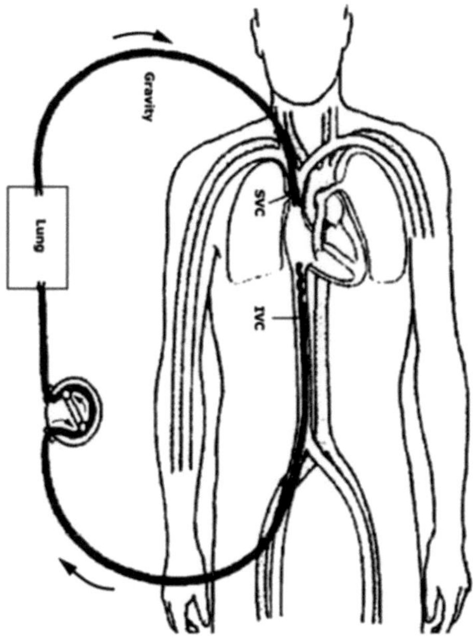

Figure 2.
Common cannulation strategy for veno-venous ECMO [75].

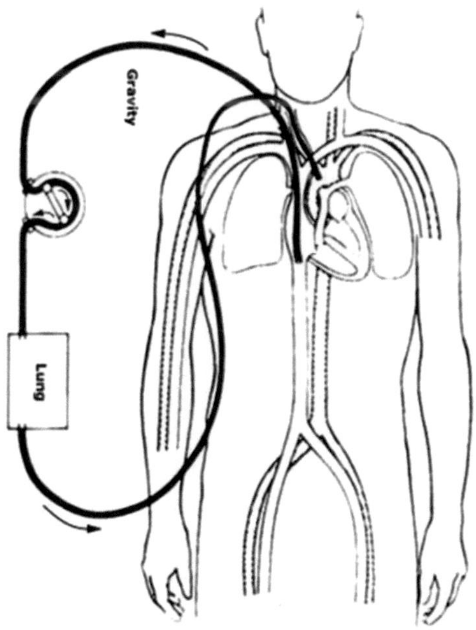

Figure 3.
Common cannulation strategy for veno-arterial ECMO [75].

Subsequently, two meta-analyses comparing the two trials showed mortality benefit for VVECMO in severe ARDS and one meta-analysis showed improvement in cardiac, renal, and neurological dysfunction (**Table 5**) [81, 82].

CESAR trial	EOLIA trial
Issues with blinding and standardization of treatment protocols. The control group did not receive uniform treatment, leading to variability in care. Some participants referred for ECMO did not receive it, affecting the study's validity [79].	Underpowering of the study. High crossover rate to ECMO in control group may have affected outcomes. Variability in ECMO implementation across centers raised concerns about consistency [80].

Table 5.
Criticisms of landmark ECMO trials [76, 77].

9.2 ESICM guidelines for ECMO in ARDS

In 2023, ESICM gave updates to their 2017 clinical practice guidelines on the management of ARDS. In their discussion on ECMO's role in ARDS, the society gave recommendations for selecting proper patient for ECMO [72]. The guidelines gave a strong recommendation for patients with severe ARDS not due to COVID-19 to be treated with ECMO with management mirroring the EOLIA trial. While noting a low level of evidence, they also extended this recommendation to patients with severe ARDS due to COVID-19 since a randomized control trial of ECMO in severe ARDS due to COVID-19 is unlikely to occur. This decision was guided by multiple observational studies in COVID-19 patients that suggested improved short-term survival with ECMO. However, the available data did not show significant differences in 0-to-90-day mortality (**Table 6**) [72].

10. Prognostication

Various prognostication models have been developed over the years. The predictive values of disease-, patient-, and management-related factors have been studied, yet none reign supreme. For example, the Murray Lung Injury Score, the PaO2/FIO2 ratio, and the Oxygenation Saturation Index [80]. Recently, two studies have tried to take another evidence-based approach to this.

In 2021, the Stratification for Identification of Prognostic Categories In the Acute RESpiratory Distress Syndrome (SPIRES) Score was formulated. SPIRES identified three variables: patient's age, number of extrapulmonary organ failures, and the PaO2/FiO2 ratio assessed at 24 hours of ARDS diagnosis. Those variables predicted ICU mortality significantly better than many previously proposed models, such as the PaO2/FiO2 ratio alone or the SOFA assessment scale [80].

In 2023, the Predicting ICU Mortality in Acute Respiratory Distress Syndrome Patients Using Machine Learning: The Predicting Outcome and STratifiCation of

Indication Criteria for ECMO in ARDS
Severe ARDS with PaO2/FIO2 < 80 mmHg for more than 6 hours
PaO2/FiO2 < 50 mmHg for more than 3 hours
pH <7.25 with PaCO2 > 60 mmHg for more than 6 hours

Table 6.
Indication criteria for ECMO in ARDS per ECISM, implemented directly from the inclusion criteria of the EOLIA trial [72].

7 Potential Predictors Identified in POSTCARDS	
• Age	• PaO_2/FIO_2 ratio
• Cancer	• Inspiratory plateau pressure
• Immunosuppression	• Number of extrapulmonary organ failures
• Baseline & 24 hr P_{plat}	

Table 7.
Predictors in POSTCARDS study [83].

severity in ARDS (POSTCARDS) Study was published. POSTCARDS used a machine learning program (MLP) and identified seven variables listed in **Table 7** with the highest predictive accuracy for 24-hour ICU mortality performance was comparable to traditional methods [83]. The POSTCARDS study did note that two different MLP did not outperform the SPIRES scoring system (AUC, 0.91; 95% CI, 0.82–0.91; SN, 0.85: SP0.84).

11. Complication, Prognosis & Long-term Outcomes

11.1 Complications

Since ARDS patients often end up requiring mechanical ventilation and intensive care unit (ICU) admission, they are at risk for VILI, nosocomial infections, such as ventilator-associated pneumonia, critical care myopathies, venous thromboembolic events, stress ulcerations, decreased nutrition and delirium [84–86]. These complications are likely multifactorial in nature; however, they lead to high morbidity and mortality in these patients.

11.2 Mortality

The Lung Safe study directly observed the outcomes of patients who had ARDS. Patients had a median duration of 8 days of ventilation, ICU stay of 10 days and total hospital stay of 17 days [84]. Mortality was directly proportional to the severity of the ARDS with 35% mortality for mild ARDS increasing up to 46% mortality for patients with severe ARDS [84–86]. Comparing ICU patients, ARDS increased mortality rate by 15% compared to those who did not have ARDS in the ICU [87]. Mortality is also increased in patients with ARDS in low-income and middle-income countries when compared to high-income countries [88]. Most of the deaths in the first 3 days are related to the underlying cause and later deaths were mostly attributed to sepsis [88, 89].

11.3 Outcomes in survivors

Among the survivors of ARDS, the cardiopulmonary function often reaches back to baseline by 6 months after the initial lung injury. Patients are, however, usually left with new or worsening cognitive, psychiatric, and physical deficits [88]. Severity of ARDS and resulting hypoxemia is associated with increased risk of cognitive deficits, including executive reasoning, verbal reasoning, memory issues and attention deficits [88]. There is an increase in depression, anxiety, and post-traumatic stress disorder (PTSD) reported in survivors [90]. The physical deficits include reduced exercise tolerance and increased disabilities, are further complicated by muscle weakness [89, 90]. There are also reports of increased hospital readmissions for up to 40% of survivors, including a third who need ICU admissions [91]. Overall, ARDS survivors experience noticeable decline in quality of life. Growing evidence shows that survivors may benefit from multidisciplinary-led post-intensive care clinics with regular intervals of follow-ups to help optimize functional status of the patient [92]. Further research is warranted into methods to improve outcomes for these patients, including the benefits of recovery programs and support groups.

12. Conclusion

Acute respiratory distress syndrome diagnosis does not adequately describe what the syndrome is. While the patient is typically in respiratory distress due to this syndrome, the diagnosis usually means acute diffuse lung injury with imaging showing bilateral infiltrates, blood gas showing severe hypoxia and/or hypercapnia while the pathology shows diffuse alveolar damage. It can portend significant morbidity and mortality. As we touched on, regardless of how ARDS is defined, and definitions are evolving, there are certain golden rules for treatment. NIV, Proning, ventilation with LTVV while keeping P_{plat} < 30 mmHg and DP <15 mmHg, steroids, restrictive fluid usage and ECMO are the usual interventions available. Our understanding of ARDS and its pathophysiology is evolving. There is increasing attention being given to ARDS phenotypes. On this front, much research remains to be done. The management and understanding of ARDS remains a dynamic and complex topic, further necessitating a multidisciplinary approach with prudent application of evidence-based strategies. Future research is likely to shift the current paradigms dramatically.

Author details

Dhaval Patel*, Moyan Sun, Sandus Khan, Schaza Javed Rana and Andrew Strike
Northeast Georgia Medical Center, Gainesville, Georgia, USA

*Address all correspondence to: dhavalpatel05@gmail.com

References

[1] Bellani G, Laffey JG, Pham T, et al. Epidemiology, patterns of care, and mortality for patients with acute respiratory distress syndrome in intensive care units in 50 countries. JAMA. 2016;**315**:788-800

[2] Martin TR, Zemans RL, Ware LB, et al. New insights into clinical and mechanistic heterogeneity of the acute respiratory distress syndrome: Summary of the Aspen lung conference 2021. American Journal of Respiratory Cell and Molccular Biology. 2022;**67**(3):284-308

[3] Matthay MA, Zemans RL, Zimmerman GA, et al. Acute respiratory distress syndrome. Nature Reviews. Disease Primers. 2019;**5**:18

[4] MacCallum NS, Evans TW. Epidemiology of acute lung injury. Current Opinion in Critical Care. 2005;**11**:43

[5] Odeyemi Y, Moraes AGD, Gajic O. What factors predispose patients to acute respiratory distress syndrome? Evidence-Based Practice of Critical Care. 2020;**103-108**:e1

[6] Beitler JR, Thompson BT, Baron RM, et al. Advancing precision medicine for acute respiratory distress syndrome. The Lancet Respiratory Medicine. 2022;**10**(1):107-120

[7] Kerchberger VE, Bastarache JA, Shaver CM, et al. Haptoglobin-2 variant increases susceptibility to acute respiratory distress syndrome during sepsis. JCI Insight. 2019;**4**(21):e131206

[8] Ware LB, Matthay MA. Alveolar fluid clearance is impaired in the majority of patients with acute lung injury and acute respiratory distress syndrome. American Journal of Respiratory and Critical Care Medicine. 2001;**163**:1376-1383

[9] Ting C, Aspal M, Vaishampayan N, et al. Fatal COVID-19 and non-COVID-19 acute respiratory distress syndrome is associated with incomplete alveolar type 1 epithelial cell differentiation from the transitional state without fibrosis. The American Journal of Pathology. 2022;**192**(3):454-467

[10] Ikegami M, Falcone A, Whitsett JA. STAT-3 regulates surfactant phospholipid homeostasis in normal lung and during endotoxin mediated lung injury. Journal of Applied Physiology. 2008;**104**:1753-1760

[11] Jansing NL, McClendon J, Henson PM, et al. Unbiased quantitation of alveolar type II to alveolar type I cell trans differentiation during repair after lung injury in mice. American Journal of Respiratory Cell and Molecular Biology. 2017;**57**:519-526

[12] Corbridge TC, Wood LDH, Crawford GP, et al. Adverse effects of large tidal volume and low PEEP in canine acid aspiration. The American Review of Respiratory Disease. 1990;**142**:311-315

[13] Marshall R, Bellingan G, Laurent G. The acute respiratory distress syndrome: Fibrosis in the fast lane. Thorax. 1998;**53**:815-817

[14] Mack M, Yanagita M. Origin of myofibroblasts and cellular events triggering fibrosis. Kidney International. 2015;**87**:297-307

[15] Prescott HC, Calfee CS, Thompson BT, et al. Toward smarter lumping and smarter splitting:

Rethinking strategies for sepsis and acute respiratory distress syndrome clinical trial design. American Journal of Respiratory and Critical Care Medicine. 2016;**194**:147-155

[16] Calfee CS, Delucchi K, Parsons PE, et al. Sub phenotypes in acute distress syndrome: Latent class analysis of data from two randomized controlled trials. The Lancet Respiratory Medicine. 2014;**2**:611-620

[17] Sinha P, Delucchi KL, Thompson BT, et al. Latent class analysis of ARDS sub phenotypes: A secondary analysis of the statins for acutely injured lungs from sepsis (SAILS) study. Intensive Care Medicine. 2018;**44**:1859-1869

[18] Constantin JM, Grasso S, Chanques G, et al. Lung morphology predicts response to recruitment maneuver in patients with acute respiratory distress syndrome. Critical Care Medicine. 2010;**38**:1108-1117

[19] Constantin JM, Jabaudon M, Lefrant J-Y, et al. Personalized mechanical ventilation tailored to lung morphology versus low positive end-expiratory pressure for patients with acute respiratory distress syndrome in France (the LIVE study): A multicenter, single blind, randomized controlled trial. The Lancet Respiratory Medicine. 2019;7:870-880

[20] The ARDS Definition Task Force*. Acute respiratory distress syndrome: The Berlin definition. Journal of the American Medical Association. 2012;**307**(23):2526-2533

[21] Matthay MA, Arabi Y, Arroliga AC, et al. A new global definition of acute respiratory distress syndrome. American Journal of Respiratory and Critical Care Medicine. 2024;**209**(1):37-47

[22] Matthay MA, Thompson BT, Ware LB. The Berlin definition of acute respiratory distress syndrome: Should patients receiving high-flow nasal oxygen be included? The Lancet Respiratory Medicine. 2021;**9**(8):933-936

[23] Figueroa-Casas JB, Brunner N, et al. Accuracy of the chest radiograph to identify bilateral pulmonary infiltrates consistent with the diagnosis of acute respiratory distress syndrome using computed tomography as reference standard. Journal of Critical Care. 2013;**28**(4):352-357

[24] Bellani G, Laffey JG, Pham T, et al. Noninvasive ventilation of patients with acute respiratory distress syndrome. Insights from the LUNG SAFE study. American Journal of Respiratory and Critical Care Medicine. 2017;**195**:67

[25] Shu W, Guo S, Yang F, et al. Association between ARDS Etiology and risk of noninvasive ventilation failure. Annals of the American Thoracic Society. 2022;**19**:255

[26] Santos C, Ferrer M, Roca J, et al. Pulmonary gas exchange response to oxygen breathing in acute lung injury. American Journal of Respiratory and Critical Care Medicine. 2000;**161**(1):26-31

[27] Butt Y, Kurdowska A, Allen TC. Acute lung injury: A clinical and molecular review. Archives of Pathology & Laboratory Medicine. 2016;**140**(4):345-350

[28] Barrot L, Asfar P, Mauny F, et al. Liberal and conservative oxygen therapy for acute respiratory distress syndrome. The New England Journal of Medicine. 2020;**382**:999

[29] Acute Respiratory Distress Syndrome Network, Brower RG, Matthay MA,

Morris A, et al. Ventilation with lower tidal volumes as compared with traditional volumes for acute lung injury and acute respiratory distress syndrome. The New England Journal of Medicine. 2000;**342**:1301

[30] Brower RG, Lanken PN, Macintyre N, et al. Higher versus lower positive end-expiratory pressures (PEEP) levels for mechanically ventilated adult patients with acute respiratory distress syndrome. The New England Journal of Medicine. 2004;**351**(4):327-336

[31] Meade MO, Cook DJ, Guyatt GH, et al. Ventilation strategy using low tidal volumes, recruitment maneuvers and high positive end expiratory pressure for acute lung injury and acute respiratory distress syndrome; a randomized control trial. JAMA. 2008;**299**:637

[32] Dianti J, Tisminetzky M, Ferreyro BL, et al. Association of Positive end-Expiratory Pressure and Lung Recruitment Selection Strategies with mortality in acute respiratory distress syndrome: A systematic review and network Meta-analysis. American Journal of Respiratory and Critical Care Medicine. 2022;**205**(11):1300-1310

[33] Santa Cruz R, Villarejo F, Irrazabal C, Ciapponi A. High versus low positive end-expiratory pressure (PEEP) levels for mechanically ventilated adult patients with acute lung injury and acute. Respiratory distress syndrome. Cochrane Database of Systematic Reviews. 2021;**2021**:CD009098

[34] Qadir N, Sahetya S, Munshi L, et al. An update on Management of Adult Patients with acute respiratory distress syndrome: An official American Thoracic Society clinical practice guideline. American Journal of Respiratory and Critical Care Medicine. 2024;**209**(1):24-36

[35] Albert RK, Jurkovich GJ, Connett J, et al. Sigh ventilation in patients with trauma. Journal of the American Medical Association. 2023;**330**(20):1982-1990

[36] Writing Group for the Alveolar Recruitment for Acute Respiratory Distress Syndrome Trial (ART) Investigators, Cavalcanti AB, Suzumura ÉA, et al. Effect of lung recruitment and titrated positive end-expiratory pressure (PEEP) vs low PEEP on mortality in patients with acute respiratory distress syndrome: A randomized clinical trial. Journal of the American Medical Association. 2017;**318**(14):1335-1345

[37] Hodgson CL, Cooper DJ, Arabi Y, et al. Maximal recruitment open lung ventilation in acute respiratory distress syndrome (PHARLAP). Phase II, Multicenter randomized controlled clinical trial. American Journal of Respiratory and Critical Care Medicine. 2019;**200**(11):1363-1372

[38] Modrykamien A, Chatburn R, Ashton R. Airway pressure release ventilation: An alternative mode of mechanical ventilation in acute respiratory distress syndrome. Cleveland Clinic Journal of Medicine. 2011;**78**:101-110

[39] Putensen C, Mutz NJ, Putensen-Himmer G, et al. Spontaneous breathing during ventilatory support improves ventilation-perfusion distributions in patients with acute respiratory distress syndrome. American Journal of Respiratory and Critical Care Medicine. 1999;**159**:1241-1248

[40] Sydow M, Burchardi H, Ephraim E, et al. Long-term effects of two different ventilatory modes on oxygenation in acute lung injury. Comparison of airway pressure release ventilation and volume-controlled inverse ratio

ventilation. American Journal of Respiratory and Critical Care Medicine. 1994;**149**:1550-1556

[41] Zhou Y, Jin X, Lv Y, et al. Early application of airway pressure release ventilation may reduce the duration of mechanical ventilation in acute respiratory distress syndrome. Intensive Care Medicine. 2017;**43**:1648-1659

[42] Amato MB, Meade MO, Slutsky AS, et al. Driving pressure and survival in acute respiratory distress syndrome. The New England Journal of Medicine. 2015;**372**:747

[43] Urner M, Jüni P, Hansen B, et al. Time-varying intensity of mechanical ventilation and mortality in patients with acute respiratory failure: A registry-based, prospective cohort study. The Lancet Respiratory Medicine. 2020;**8**(9):905-913

[44] Gattinoni L, Tonetti T, Cressoni M, et al. Ventilator-related causes of lung injury: The mechanical power. Intensive Care Medicine. 2016;**42**:1567-1575

[45] Van der Meijden S et al. Calculating mechanical power for pressure-controlled ventilation. Intensive Care Medicine. 2019;**45**:1495-1497

[46] Chiumello D, Gotti M, Guanziroli M, et al. Bedside calculation of mechanical power during volume- and pressure-controlled mechanical ventilation. Critical Care. 2020;*24*:417

[47] Rietveld PJ et al. Mechanical power differs between pressure-controlled ventilation and different volume-controlled ventilation modes. Critical Care Explorations. 2022;**4**(8):e0741

[48] Slutsky AS, Ranieri VM. Ventilator-induced lung injury. The New England Journal of Medicine. 2013;**369**(22):2126-2136

[49] Beitler JR, Malhotra A, Thompson BT. Ventilator-induced lung injury. Clinics in Chest Medicine. 2016;**37**(4):633-646

[50] De Durante G, del Turco M, Rustichini L, et al. ARDSNet lower tidal volume ventilatory strategy may generate intrinsic positive and expiratory pressure in patients with acute respiratory distress syndrome. American Journal of Respiratory and Critical Care Medicine. 2002;**165**:1271

[51] Kahn JM, Andersson L, Karitr V, et al. Low tidal volume ventilation does not increase sedation use in patients with acute lung injury. Critical Care Medicine. 2005;**33**:766

[52] Thile AW, Rodriguez P, Cabello B, et al. Patient-ventilator asynchrony during assisted mechanical ventilation. Intensive Care Medicine. 2006;**32**:1515

[53] Tobin MJ, Jubran A, Laghi F. Patient-ventilator interaction. American Journal of Respiratory and Critical Care Medicine. 2001;**163**:1059

[54] De Wit M, Pedram S, Best AM, et al. Observational study of patient ventilator asynchrony and relationship to sedation level. Journal of Critical Care. 2009;**24**:74

[55] Akoumianiki E, Lyazidi A, Rey N, et al. Mechanical ventilation-induced reverse-triggered breaths: A frequently unrecognized form of neuromechanical coupling. Chest. 2013;**143**:927

[56] National Heart, Lung, and Blood Institute Acute Respiratory Distress Syndrome (ARDS) Clinical Trials Network, Wiedemann HP, Wheeler AP, et al. Comparison of two fluid-management strategies in acute

lung injury. The New England Journal of Medicine. 2006;**354**(24):2564-2575

[57] Grissom CK, Hirshberg EL, Dickerson JB, et al. Fluid management with a simplified conservative protocol for the acute respiratory distress syndrome*. Critical Care Medicine. 2015;**43**(2):288-295

[58] Liu X, Jiang Y, Jia X, et al. Identification of distinct clinical phenotypes of acute respiratory distress syndrome with differential responses to treatment. Critical Care. 2021;**25**(1):320

[59] Lai-Fook SJ, Rodarte JR. Pleural pressure distribution and its relationship to lung volume and interstitial pressure. Journal of Applied Physiology. 1985;**70**(3):967-978

[60] Cornejo RA, Díaz JC, Tobar EA, et al. Effects of prone positioning on lung protection in patients with acute respiratory distress syndrome. American Journal of Respiratory and Critical Care Medicine. 2013;**188**(4):440-448

[61] Guérin C, Albert RK, Beitler J, et al. Prone position in ARDS patients: Why, when how and for whom. Intensive Care Medicine. 2020;**46**:2385-2396

[62] Langer M, Mascheroni D, Marcolin R, Gattinoni L. The prone position in ARDS patients. A clinical study. Chest. 1988;**94**(1):103-107

[63] Munshi L, Del Sorbo L, Adhikari NKJ, et al. Prone position for acute respiratory distress syndrome. A systematic review and Meta-analysis. Annals of the American Thoracic Society. 2017;**14**:S280

[64] Gattinoni L, Tognoni G, Pesenti A, et al. Effect of prone positioning on the survival of patients with acute respiratory failure. The New England Journal of Medicine. 2001;**345**(8):568-573

[65] Qian ET, Gatto CL, Amusina O, et al. Assessment of awake prone positioning in hospitalized adults with COVID-19: A nonrandomized controlled trial. JAMA Internal Medicine. 2022;**182**(6):612-621

[66] Li J, Luo J, Pavlov I, et al. Awake prone positioning for non-intubated patients with COVID-19-related acute hypoxaemic respiratory failure: A systematic review and meta-analysis. The Lancet Respiratory Medicine. 2022;**10**(6):573-583

[67] Schmidt M, Hajage D, Lebreton G, et al. Prone positioning during extracorporeal membrane oxygenation in patients with severe ARDS: The PRONECMO randomized clinical trial. JAMA. 2023;**330**(24):2343-2353

[68] Villar J, Ferrando C, Martínez D, et al. Dexamethasone treatment for the acute respiratory distress syndrome: A multicentre, randomised controlled trial. The Lancet Respiratory Medicine. 2020;**8**(3):267-276

[69] Zhou Y, Fu X, Liu X, et al. Use of corticosteroids in influenza-associated acute respiratory distress syndrome and severe pneumonia: A systemic review and meta-analysis. Scientific Reports. 2020;**10**(1):3044

[70] Papazian L, Forel JM, Gacouin A, et al. Neuromuscular blockers in early acute respiratory distress syndrome. The New England Journal of Medicine. 2010;**363**(12):1107-1116

[71] National Heart, Lung, and Blood Institute PETAL Clinical Trials Network, Moss M, Huang DT, et al. Early neuromuscular blockade in the acute respiratory distress syndrome.

The New England Journal of Medicine. 2019;**380**(21):1997-2008

[72] Grasselli G, Calfee CS, Camporota L, et al. ESICM guidelines on acute respiratory distress syndrome: Definition, phenotyping and respiratory support strategies. Intensive Care Medicine. 2023;**49**(7):727-759

[73] Liaqat A, Mason M, Foster BJ, Kulkarni S, Barlas A, Farooq AM, et al. Evidence-based mechanical ventilatory strategies in ARDS. Journal of Clinical Medicine. 2022;**11**(2):319

[74] Fanelli V, Giani M, Grasselli G, et al. Extracorporeal membrane oxygenation for COVID-19 and influenza H1N1 associated acute respiratory distress syndrome: A multicenter retrospective cohort study. Critical Care. 2022;**26**(1):34

[75] Van Meurs K, Lally KP, Peek G, Zwischenberger JB. ECMO Extracorporeal Cardiopulmonary Support in Critical Care. Ann Arbor, MI: Extracorporeal Life Support Organization; 2005. p. 290

[76] Peek GJ, Clemens F, Elbourne D, et al. CESAR: Conventional ventilatory support vs extracorporeal membrane oxygenation for severe adult respiratory failure. BMC Health Services Research. 2006;**6**:163

[77] Sameed M, Meng Z, Marciniak ET. EOLIA trial: The future of extracorporeal membrane oxygenation in acute respiratory distress syndrome therapy? Breathe (Sheffield, England). 2019;**15**(3):244-246

[78] Goligher EC, Tomlinson G, Hajage D, et al. Extracorporeal membrane oxygenation for severe acute respiratory distress syndrome and posterior probability of mortality benefit in a post hoc Bayesian analysis of a randomized clinical trial. Journal of the American Medical Association. 2018;**320**(21):2251-2259

[79] Gattinoni L, Vasques F, Quintel M. Use of ECMO in ARDS: Does the EOLIA trial really help? Critical Care. 2018;**22**(1):171

[80] Villar J, González-Martín JM, Ambrós A, et al. Stratification for identification of prognostic categories in the acute RESpiratory distress syndrome (SPIRES) score. Critical Care Medicine. 2021;**49**(10):e920-e930

[81] Combes A et al. ECMO for severe ARDS: Systematic review and individual patient data meta-analysis. Intensive Care Medicine. 2020;**46**(11):2048-2057

[82] Vaquer S et al. Systematic review and meta-analysis of complications and mortality of veno-venous extracorporeal membrane oxygenation for refractory acute respiratory distress syndrome. Annals of Intensive Care. 2017;**7**(1):51

[83] Villar J, González-Martín JM, Hernández-González J, et al. Predicting ICU mortality in acute respiratory distress syndrome patients using machine learning: The predicting outcome and STratifiCation of severity in ARDS (POSTCARDS) study. Critical Care Medicine. 2023;**51**(12):1638-1649

[84] Bellani G, Laffey JG, Pham T, et al. Epidemiology, patterns of care, and mortality for patients with acute respiratory distress syndrome in intensive care units in 50 countries. JAMA. 2016;**315**:788

[85] Fagon JY, Chastre J, Vuagnat A, et al. Nosocomial pneumonia and mortality among patients in intensive care units. JAMA. 1996;**275**:866

[86] McNicoll L, Pisani MA, Zhang Y, et al. Delirium in the intensive care unit:

Occurrence and clinical course in older patients. Journal of the American Geriatrics Society. 2003;**51**:591

[87] Torres LK, Hoffman KL, Oromendia C, et al. Attributable mortality of acute respiratory distress syndrome: A systematic review, metaanalysis and survival analysis using targeted minimum loss-based estimation. Thorax. 2021;**76**:1176-1185

[88] Gupta E, Hossen S, Grigsby MR, et al. Risk factors for the development of acute respiratory distress syndrome in mechanically ventilated adults in Peru: A multicenter observational study. Critical Care. 2019;**23**:398

[89] Fazzini B, Battaglini D, Carenzo L, et al. Physical and psychological impairment in survivors of acute respiratory distress syndrome: A systematic review and meta-analysis. British Journal of Anaesthesia. 2022;**129**:801

[90] Bienvenu OJ, Colantuoni E, Mendez-Tellez PA, et al. Depressive symptoms and impaired physical function after acute lung injury: A 2-year longitudinal study. American Journal of Respiratory and Critical Care Medicine. 2012;**185**:517

[91] Ruhl AP, Huang M, Colantuoni E, et al. Healthcare utilization and costs in ARDS survivors: A 1-year longitudinal national US multicenter study. Intensive Care Medicine. 2017;**43**:980-991

[92] McPeake J, Iwashyna TJ, Boehm LM, et al. Benefits of peer support for intensive care unit survivors: Sharing experiences, care debriefing, and altruism. American Journal of Critical Care. 2021;**30**:145-149

Chapter 5

Role of Amikacin in the Management of Ventilator-Associated Pneumonia

Abdul Moeed, Zoha Bilal, Fizzah Batool, Asma Batool Zaidi, Muhammad Arsalan Jamil and Salim Surani

Abstract

Ventilator-associated pneumonia accounts for 60% of healthcare-associated infection deaths. It results from invasion of the lower respiratory tract by microorganisms and affects patients 48 hours after they have been intubated and have received mechanical ventilation. Prompt diagnosis using a combination of clinical, radiographic, microbiological, and laboratory assessment can help prevent exacerbation of symptoms and provide immediate treatment. Usage of antibiotics for therapy has proven clinically useful; however, emerging resistance of microorganisms to these medications has been continuously evolving. This article focuses on amikacin and how its emerging role in treating VAP has improved patient outcomes and increased their chances of recovery with minimal adverse effects.

Keywords: amikacin, antibiotics, management, ventilator-associated pneumonia, hospital-acquiredds

1. Introduction

Ventilator-associated events (VAEs) are mainly caused due to pneumonia, fluid overload, ARDS, and atelactasis, and about 40% of ventilator-associated pneumonias (VAP) meet the criteria for VAE [1]. VAP manifests as pneumonia occurring more than 48 hours subsequent to patients undergoing intubation and mechanical ventilation. An overwhelming 86% of all hospital-acquired pneumonias are linked to mechanical ventilation, with VAP's mortality rates fluctuating between 0 and 50%, contingent upon the specific pathogens identified. When specifying areas of the hospital most affected by VAP, a study by Song et al. showed that there was no true difference seen between the incidence of VAP in medical intensive care units(MICU) when compared to surgical intensive care units(SICU), neither was there a significant difference in mortalities ($P = 0.228$); however, the length of stay for MICU patients with VAP was significantly prolonged as compared to those who had not contracted VAP, averaging on 6 and 8.5 days, respectively ($P < 0.001$) [2]. Hence, apart from its medical implications, VAP also imposes significant financial burdens on patients due to prolonged hospital stays. Furthermore, effective treatment necessitates diligent nursing care, respiratory therapy, and prudent antibiotic administration.

Selecting the appropriate therapy for VAP mandates adherence to certain principles, including awareness of prevalent organisms, local resistance patterns within the ICU, a rationale for antibiotic selection, and considerations for de-escalation or cessation of antibiotic therapy. Studies have underscored the criticality of timely initiation of appropriate antibiotic treatment for VAP, as delays have been correlated with increased mortality rates.

In case of absence of risk factors for multidrug-resistant bacteria, clinicians typically opt for empirical therapy targeting *Streptococcus pneumoniae*, methicillin-sensitive *Staphylococcus aureus*, *Haemophilus influenzae*, and susceptible gram-negative enteric organisms [3]. This empirical regimen typically comprises an antipseudomonal cephalosporin (such as cefepime or ceftazidime), an antipseudomonal carbapenem (such as imipenem or meropenem), or a β-lactam/β-lactamase inhibitor (such as piperacillin-tazobactam), coupled with an aminoglycoside (such as amikacin or gentamicin) or an antipseudomonal fluoroquinolone (like ciprofloxacin or levofloxacin). Recent research has highlighted the potential efficacy of inhaled antibiotics, particularly amikacin. This chapter aims to delve deeper into this aspect [4].

1.1 Pathogenesis

With the increasing burden of disease and ICU admissions, understanding the development and pathogenesis of ventilator-associated pneumonia (VAP) is crucial for devising effective treatment strategies.

Microorganisms causing VAP must first access the normally sterile lower respiratory tract, where they adhere to the mucosa and establish infection. There are four primary mechanisms through which microorganisms gain access: aspiration of microbe-laden secretions from the oropharynx, direct extension from contiguous infections, inhalation of contaminated air or medical aerosols, and hematogenous carriage from remote infection site [5].

In non-intubated patients, the oropharyngeal flora primarily consists of viridans streptococci, Haemophilus species, and anaerobes, maintained by factors like the flow and content of saliva. However, in critically ill patients, especially in ICUs, there's a significant shift toward aerobic gram-negative bacilli and *Staphylococcus aureus* [6]. Various factors such as reduced mucosal immunoglobulin A, increased protease production, and altered airway receptors contribute to bacterial adherence to the orotracheal mucosa in mechanically ventilated patients.

Aspiration of oropharyngeal contents overwhelms compromised host defenses, leading to VAP development. The stomach serves as a potential reservoir for VAP-causing bacteria [7], particularly in conditions like elevated gastric pH due to factors such as treatment with acid-suppressing medications or enteral nutrition. Gastric microorganisms can reflux up the esophagus and are aspirated into the trachea, implicating the stomach in VAP development.

Furthermore, the endotracheal tube (ETT) acts as a conduit for microbial colonization, providing a direct route for bacteria to bypass upper respiratory tract defenses. Biofilm formation on the ETT surface further facilitates bacterial adhesion and colonization, promoting the persistence of infection despite antimicrobial therapy.

Ventilator-induced lung injury (VILI) plays a significant role in VAP pathogenesis. Mechanical ventilation disrupts the normal physiological mechanisms of airway clearance and immune defense, leading to impaired mucociliary clearance [8], reduced cough reflex, and compromised alveolar macrophage function. Additionally, high tidal volumes and positive end-expiratory pressure (PEEP) can cause barotrauma and volutrauma, resulting in lung tissue damage and inflammation, which further predisposes the lung to infection.

In summary, VAP pathogenesis is multifactorial, involving microbial colonization facilitated by the endotracheal tube, disruption of normal lung defense mechanisms by mechanical ventilation, and dysregulation of the host immune response. Understanding these intricate processes is essential for developing targeted preventive strategies and optimizing management approaches to reduce the burden of VAP in critically ill patients.

In understanding the intricate processes of VAP pathogenesis, we are better equipped to develop targeted preventive strategies and optimize management approaches. Now, let us delve into the crucial aspect of diagnosing VAP to ensure timely and effective interventions for improving patient outcomes.

1.2 Diagnosis of VAP

VAP requires the implementation of multiple clinical manifestations for its prompt diagnosis. The recommended diagnostic measures are as follows: (i) radiographic assessment (manifestation of new or progressive lung infiltrates and consolidation or cavitation); (ii) laboratory assessment (white blood cell count >4 or at least 12×10^3 cells/mm^3); (iii) clinical assessment (such as a body temperature < 36°C or > 38°C, new onset or increase of purulent aspirates, wheezing, rales, rhonchi, or progressive worsening of gas exchange); (iv) microbiological criteria (showcasing positive culture result from suctioned sputum, bronchoscopy, blind bronchoalveolar lavage, or pleural fluid) [9–11]. Several criteria have been proposed for diagnosing VAP in clinical settings, which is summarized in the **Table 1**.

The National Nosocomial Infection Surveillance (NNIS) system, developed in the 1970s by the Centers for Disease Control (CDC), was implemented to study the distribution of hospital acquired infections. It was compared to 292 bronchoalveolar lavage (BAL) fluid cultures obtained from trauma patients and was found to have a sensitivity of 84% and a specificity of 69% [12].

Subsequently, Pugin et al. [13]. proposed the Clinical Pulmonary Infection Score (CPIS), which takes into account the following six variables: fever, white blood cell count, tracheal aspirates, oxygenation of the blood, radiographic consolidation, and semiquantitative cultures of tracheal aspirates using Gram stain. This criterion originally showed 93% sensitivity and 100% specificity; however, it only included results from 28 patients. Along with that, the results were compared to quantitative cultures of BAL fluid using a bacterial index (sum of the logarithm of all bacterial species recovered), which cannot be accounted for as an acceptable gold standard for diagnosis of VAP.

When compared to a pathological diagnosis, CPIS showed sensitivity between 72 and 77% and specificity between 42 and 85% [14, 15]. Pham et al. [16]. compared quantitative BAL fluid culture to diagnose VAP and concluded that CPIS had a sensitivity of 30% and specificity of 80%.

Johnson et al. [17] suggested that diagnosis of VAP should be made by onset of a new or worsening consolidation in chest radiology along with evidence of any two of the following variables: fever >38°C, increased white blood cell count, and purulent secretions. When Fabregas et al. [14]. chose to compare immediate post-mortem lung biopsies, its sensitivity was only 69%, and specificity reached 75%, proving this criterion to have low accuracy. Despite this relatively low accuracy, these criteria were approved by the American Thoracic Society Consensus Conference for correct diagnosis of VAP [18].

VAP is also classified based on the onset of symptoms. Development in less than 4 days of admission is considered early-onset VAP, and it most commonly arises as a

Clinical criteria used in diagnosing ventilator-associated pneumonia		
Johnson criteria	**Clinical Pulmonary Infection Score (CPIS)**	**Centers for Disease Control and Prevention (CDC)**
• Presence of a new or progressive radiographic infiltrate	• Temperature • 0 point: 36.5–38.4 C • 1 point: 38.5–38.9 • 2 points: < 36 or > 39 • Oxygenation (PaO2/FiO2) • 0 point: PaO2/FiO2 > 240 or ARDS • 2 points: PaO2/FiO2 < 240 and no ARDS	• Radiology signs Two or more serial chest radiographs with at least 1 of the following: • new or progressive and persistent infiltrate • consolidation • cavitation
• Plus at least two of three clinical features: • fever >38°C • leukocytosis or leukopenia • purulent secretions	• Tracheal secretions (score) • 0 point: < 14 • 1 point: > 14 • 2 points: purulent sputum • Culture of tracheal aspirate • 0 point: minimal or no growth • 1 point: moderate or more growth • 2 points: moderate or greater growth	• Microbiological criteria At least one of the following: • positive growth in blood culture unrelated to any previous infection • growth seen in culture or pleural field • positive quantitative culture from bronchoalveolar lavage $(>10^4)$ or protected specimen brushing $(>10^3)$ • 5% or more of cells with intracellular bacteria on direct microscopic examination of Gram-stained BAL fluid • histopathological evidence of presence of pneumonia
	• Blood leukocytes (cells/μL) • 0 point: 4000–11,000 • 1 point: < 4000 or > 11,000 • 2 points: > 500 band forms • Pulmonary radiography • 0 point: no infiltrate • 1 point: diffuse or patchy infiltrates • 2 points: localized infiltrate	• Clinical signs At least 1 of the following: • fever (temperature > 38°C) • leukopenia (< 4000 WBC) or leukocytosis (> 12,000 WBC) • altered mental status seen in adults over the age of 70 with no other recognized cause Plus at least 2 of the following: • onset of newly developed purulent sputum, or change in character and quality of sputum • increased respiratory secretions within the lung, or increased suctioning requirements seen • onset of any of the following: worsening cough, dyspnea, tachypnea • bronchial sounds or rales • progressive worsening of gas exchange • increased oxygen requirements for the body
	Total score of >6 points suggests ventilator-associated pneumonia	

Table 1.
Criteria for diagnosis of ventilator-associated pneumonia.

result of microorganisms sensitive to antibiotics. On the other hand, development of VAP more than 4 days after admission is classified as late-onset VAP and is usually due to MDR pathogens [9].

Delayed diagnosis, along with a delay in its required therapy, may lead to worsening symptoms in patients with VAP. Similarly, a false diagnosis will lead to unwarranted treatment and its associated complications. An early and clinically accurate diagnosis is key in managing patients with VAP [16].

1.3 Management of VAP

Current guidelines prepared by a joint committee of American Thoracic Society (ATS) and Infectious Diseases Society of America (IDSA) consider late-onset VAP a risk for MDR pathogens, so they aim to focus more on identification of risk factors and prompt administration of empiric therapy so as to not exacerbate symptoms.

Pathogens that are most often seen to be causing VAP include gram-negative bacteria such as *P. aeruginosa*, *Escherichia coli*, *Acinetobacter* species, *K. pneumoniae*, and Gram-positive bacteria such as Staphylococcus aureus [9].

Antibiotics that target specific pathogens of VAP are ideally recommended for treatment of clinically suspected VAP to allow for coverage of *Staphylococcus aureus*, *Pseudomonas aeruginosa*, and other gram-negative bacilli so as to minimize overtreatment and its subsequent outcomes. The **Table 2** summarizes different treatment modalities for VAP proposed over the years.

Guideline	Empiric treatment recommendation	Aerosolized antibiotic recommendation	Duration of antibiotic therapy
Qiu [19]	—	For VAP/HAP patients infected with gram-negative bacteria, that is, identified as multidrug-resistant, a combination of systemic antibiotics and aerosol inhalation antibiotics can be considered to improve the cure and clearance rate of respiratory bacteria responsible for causing pneumonia.	—
Qu [20]	For HAP/VAP patients with risk factors of MDR Pseudomonas aeruginosa and other MDR gram-negative bacilli infection or high risk of death, the combination of two different types of antibiotics is recommended. HAP/VAP patients who are not critical/have no risk factors for MDR infection can be given a single antibiotic as empirical treatment	—	—

Guideline	Empiric treatment recommendation	Aerosolized antibiotic recommendation	Duration of antibiotic therapy
	—	The administration of nebulized colimycin (sodium colistimethate) and/or aminoglycosides is suggested; the suggested treatment as multidrug-resistant gram-negative bacilli are proven to be sensitive to the aforementioned drug combination when no other antibiotics are being used	The recommended duration for antibiotic treatment in the case of HAP should be less than 7 days except during specific situations like immunosuppression, empyema, necrotizing or abscessed pneumonia
Torres et al, [5]	It may be advisable to base empiric treatment plans on local prevalence of pathogens linked to VAP and their susceptibility to antibiotics.	—	Using a 7–8-day course of antibiotic therapy is suggested in VAP patients who are not diagnosed with immunodeficiency, cystic fibrosis, empyema, lung abscess, cavitation, or necrotizing pneumonia and having a good clinical response to therapy
Kalil [21]	It may be advisable to base empiric treatment plans on local prevalence of pathogens linked to VAP and their susceptibility to antibiotics.	Patients that are known to have been infected by gram-negative bacilli leading to VAP, which are susceptible only to aminoglycoside or polymyxins, are advised to receive both inhaled and systemic antibiotics, as opposed to just systemic antibiotics alone	For patients with VAP, a 7-day course of antimicrobial therapy rather than a longer duration is recommended

Table 2.
Guidelines for the management of ventilator-associated pneumonia.

1.4 Empirical antibiotics

Twenty-one recommendations on empiric therapy for treatment of VAP were gathered from a compilation of four guidelines [5, 18, 22, 23]. All the guidelines advised for the implementation of an empirical treatment plan are based on local prevalence of pathogens linked to VAP and their susceptibility to antibiotics. Due to this, narrow-spectrum antibiotics such as ertapenem, cefotaxime, moxifloxacin, or levofloxacin were recommended for patients with a lower likelihood of developing multidrug resistance (MDR) infection and early-onset VAP [23].

Antibiotic combination therapy was considered suitable if the pathogen was considered empirically to be multidrug resistant. The 2016 guidelines from the Infectious Diseases Society of America (IDSA) [24] recommended empirical dual therapy targeting both gram-negative bacteria and MRSA, with vancomycin or linezolid as the standard suggested treatment.

1.5 Etiological treatment

Fifteen recommendations on etiological treatment for VAP were gathered. Once the infecting pathogen is identified, its corresponding antimicrobial treatment plan should be administered with reference to the results obtained from *in vitro* drug sensitivity tests. This detailed treatment plan can be seen in the IDSA 2016 guideline [24], CMA 2018 guideline [24], and IDST 2018 guideline [21]; however, the CMA 2018 guideline and IDST 2018 guideline did not give any recommendations on strength.

The 2016 JAID guideline [21] recommendeds sulbactam (SBT) and ampicillin (ABPC) as the first-choice drug for respiratory infections caused by Acinetobacter Baumann. The CMA 2018 guideline also recommends SBT in combination with polymyxin, tigecycline, or doxycycline. However, the IDSA 2016 guideline warned against the use of tigecycline for patients with VAP caused by Acinobacter species, since it was related to worsening of outcomes compared with other therapies.

2. Aerosol inhalation antibiotic therapy

Four guidelines [5, 25–27] recommend aerosol inhalation antibiotic therapy for the treatment of VAP, while the 2018 CMA guidelines reinforce improved cure rate and clearance rate of respiratory bacteria causing pneumonia for patients infected with multi-drug resistant gram-negative bacteria.

2.1 Duration of antibiotic treatment

The IDSA 2016 guideline and SFAR 2018 guidelines [27] strongly recommend a 7-day course of antimicrobial treatment, while the ERS 2017 guideline [28] weakly recommends a 7–8-day course of antibiotic therapy. The IDSA 2016 guideline reported a decrease in antibiotic exposure and antibiotic resistance without increasing mortality or recurrent disease, hence reducing cost and side effects.

Timely commencement of management and appropriate dosage of therapy are crucial for critically ill patients to ensure adequate treatment and reduction of morbidity and mortality. Over the years, various antibiotic therapies have been used to treat VAP based on isolated microorganisms.

Active agents against methicillin-resistant *Staphylococcus aureus* like vancomycin and linezolid have been used to treat VAP in patients with antimicrobial resistance. However, based on current research, the most effective antimicrobial agents against *P. aeruginosa* are antipseudomonal antibiotics. They can be further classified into β-lactams (ticarcillin, piperacillin, aztreonam, imipenem, cefsulodin, cefoperazone, and ceftazidime), non–β-lactams (like ciprofloxacin, levofloxacin, amikacin, gentamicin, tobramycin, colistin, polymyxin), and most recent aminoglycosides, fluoroquinolones, and fosfomycin. The combination of ceftazidime and amikacin is regarded as the primary treatment plan for antipseudomonal chemotherapy [29]. **Table 3** reflects the different antibiotic groups used against various organisms.

Drug	Spectrum	Labeled indications
Ceftobiprole	Nonextended spectrum β-lactamase, non-AmpC, and non-carbapenemases-producing *Enterobacterales*, *P. aeruginosa*, MRSA	EMA: HAP excluding VAP, CAP, ABSSSI
Ceftazidime-avibactam	ESBL, KPC, AmpC, and some OXA (e.g., OXA 48)-producing *Enterobacterales*, MDR *P. aeruginosa*, MDR *A. baumannii*	FDA: HAP/VAP, cUTIs, cIAIs EMA: all those infections due to aerobic gram-negative organisms with limited treatment options
Ceftolozane-tazobactam	ESBL-producing *Enterobacterales*, MDR *P. aeruginosa*, some anaerobes, *Streptococcus* spp., MSSA	FDA: HAP/VAP, cUTIs, cIAIs EMA: HAP/VAP, cUTIs, cIAIs
Meropenem-vaborbactam	ESBL, KPC, AmpC-producing *Enterobacterales*, non-MDR *P. aeruginosa*, non-MDR *A. baumannii*, *Streptococcus* spp. MSSA	FDA: cUTI, including pyelonephritis. EMA: cUTI (including pyelonephritis), HAP, VAP, cIAI, and infections due to aerobic GNB with limited treatment options
Imipenem-relebactam cilastatin	ESBL, KPC-producing *Enterobacterales*, MDR *P. aeruginosa*, *Streptococcus* spp., MSSA	FDA: HAP/VAP, cIAI, cUTI; EMA: infections due to aerobic GNB with limited or no other therapeutic options
Cefiderocol	ESBL, CRE (class A, B, and D enzymes), CR *P. aeruginosa, S. maltophilia, A. baumannii, Streptococcus* spp.	FDA: cUTI, HAP/VAP EMA: infections due to aerobic GNB with limited therapeutic options

Table 3.
Different antibiotics used for different organisms causing ventilator-associated pneumonia.

3. Ceftolozane-tazobactam

Ceftolozane-tazobactam is a combination of a fifth-generation cephalosporin with a β-lactamase inhibitor. Ceftolozane is capable of overcoming bacterial resistance, and using it in combination with tazobactam expands its activity against β-lactamases-producing Enterobacterales [30]. During *in vitro* studies, ceftolozane–tazobactam shows increased activity against *P. aeruginosa*, since it is more active against MDR or extremely drug-resistant (XDR) strains [31] A multicenter Italian cohort study included 101 patients treated with ceftolozane–tazobactam for severe infections caused by *P. aeruginosa*. Overall, 84 patients showed clinical success out of 101 (83.2%) after treatment. A clinical success rate of 75% was also seen in the subgroup of nosocomial pneumonia [32].

3.1 Meropenem-vaborbactam

Meropenem–vaborbactam is a β-lactamase inhibitor combined with a carbapenem made with the intention of exhibiting high activity against MDR Enterobacterales [33].

The *in vitro* activity of meropenem–vaborbactam against gram-negative isolates was tested on hospitalized patients with pneumonia, including VAP, which showed the highest susceptibility rates against Enterobacterales isolates (98.0%). Along with this, meropenem–vaborbactam was seen as the most active β-lactam tested (82.1% susceptible) against *P. aeruginosa* isolates, with amikacin (86.0%) and colistin (99.4%) showing higher susceptibility rates [34].

3.2 Imipenem-relebactam

Imipenem is a cabapenem antibiotic that is used in combination with relebactam, a bicyclic diazabicyclooctane β-lactamase inhibitor. The addition of relebactam to imipenem increases the activity of the carbapenem against gram-negative bacteria, including strains that are not susceptible to imipenem such as P. aeruginosa and some β-lactamase-producing Enterobacterales [29]. The rate of sensitivity of P. aeruginosa to imipenem–relebactam was approximately 90% [35].

3.3 Cefiderocol

Cefiderocol is a cephalosporin that exhibits activity against gram-negative bacilli, including Enterobacterales, allowing it to remain stable in the presence of all classes of β-lactamases. A CREDIBLE-CR study trial was carried out to compare cefiderocol with BAT for treating HAP, VAP, cUTI, or bloodstream infections due to carbapenem-resistant gram-negative bacilli.

Nosocomial pneumonia was present in 15% of the patients, and almost 25% of them were diagnosed with VAP. The most common isolates found from this test were *A. baumannii* (46%, 54 patients), *K. pneumoniae* (33%, 39 patients), and *P. aeruginosa* (19%, 22 patients).

Regarding patients with HAP and VAP who were infected by *A. baumannii*, mortality was seen to be much higher in the cefiderocol group (42%) when compared with the BAT group (18%) [36].

3.4 Amikacin in VAP

Timely commencement of management and appropriate dosage of therapy are crucial for critically ill patients to ensure adequate treatment and reduce morbidity and mortality. Over the years, various antibiotic therapies have been used and are still used to treat VAP based on the microorganism isolated [37].

Amikacin is an aminoglycoside that targets more resistant gram-negative bacilli causing VAP, such as Acinetobacter baumanii and *Pseudomonas aeruginosa*, which are some of the most difficult nosocomial infections to treat. Amikacin kills bacteria by binding to the 30S bacterial ribosome subunit, which interferes with a reading of the genetic code and hence inhibits protein synthesis by, for example, eliciting premature protein termination and incorporating incorrect amino acid resulting in insufficient protein synthesis for the survival of the microorganism. Over the years, amikacin has been used increasingly and has shown good outcomes in treating VAP.

Amikacin is widely used in two forms—intravenous and nebulized. Initially, it was used in its IV form alongside medications such as carbapenems, cephalosporins, penicillins, and beta-lactamase inhibitors [38]. Introduction of amikacin to treatment guidelines dramatically altered care of patients in ICUs for the better, particularly in hospitals with high gentamicin and tobramycin resistance. Of 2661 gram-negative isolated in a study, an estimate of 2.0% were found to be resistant to gentamicin, while only 1.3% were resistant to amikacin [39]. This is because amikacin reduces the inactivation of bacterial acetylase, adenylase, and phosphorylase relatively more than other aminoglycosides [40].

However, the recent introduction of nebulized form of amikacin has revolutionized treatment and prevention of VAP in critically ill patients. When aerosolized amikacin was combined with IV forms of the antibiotics listed earlier, it showed to improve patient outcomes and increased chances of recovery. In order to prove this, a trial was done on 90 patients with VAP who were categorized randomly into three equal groups: Group I received IV amikacin and meropenem. Group II received the same as Group I with nebulized amikacin. Group III received IV amikacin, nebulized amikacin, and meropenem. Groups II and III showed a higher cure rate (53.33% and 66.67%, respectively) compared to Group I (26.67%, $P = 0.007$). Group II showed relatively significant reduction in ventilator days (5.32 ± 1.86 vs. 7.3 ± 2.1 days, respectively, $P < 0.001$) and reduction in ICU stay (11.87 ± 2.6 vs. 15.3 ± 3.1 days, respectively, $P < 0.001$) compared to Group I. Group III showed significant reduction in days of ventilation (4.22 ± 1.32 vs. 5.32 ± 1.86, respectively, $P = 0.011$) and a particularly significant reduction in ICU stay (9.21 ± 1.17 vs. 11.87 ± 2.6, respectively, $P < 0.001$) compared to Group II [41].

A combination of nebulized and IV amikacin is also a combination frequently used. A 5-year observational study was conducted, which had 154 patients diagnosed with VAP caused by P aeruginosa, who were split into two categories: (i) 79 consecutive patients treated with IV amikacin from January 2011 to August 2013, and (ii) 75 consecutive patients received nebulized amikacin administered from September 2013 to February 2016. In both groups, amikacin was taken for 1 to 5 days with an IV β-lactam for 10–14 days. Results showed that the aerosol group had a clinical cure rate of 72%, while the IV group showed 58%, with a significant difference of $p = 0.02$ between the two groups. This proves the significance of nebulized amikacin in treatment of VAP, and it does so by providing better oxygenation and organism clearance by allowing more product to reach the site of infection, that is, the lungs [42].

Additional benefits to using aerosolized forms of amikacin are that it has even proven to cause fewer side effects like nephrotoxicity and lessens the duration of mechanical ventilation and ICU stay. A recent study was carried out on 64 mechanically ventilated patients with gram-negative VAP. The patients were divided into two groups: Group A was treated with nebulized amikacin plus IV amikacin and included 32 patients, while 32 patients in group B were treated with IV amikacin alone. Both groups were given treatment for a duration of 8 days. The results of this study showed that Group A had a significant improvement of oxygenation before and after treatment (p 0.006), compared to group B that showed no significant difference (p 0.212). The length of stay was 21.5 days in Group A and 25.5 days in Group B, with a relatively significant reduction in group A (p 0.037). The duration of mechanical ventilation in Group A of 19 days was much less than Group B that showed 23 days, with a significant reduction (p 0.045) of ventilator days.

Additionally, Group B showed a significant rise of creatinine level after treatment ($p < 0.001$), while no significant rise in creatinine level was found in Group A after treatment. A noteworthy difference between groups A and B (p 0.003) was also seen after the end of treatment. The mortality was 19 (60%) in Group A and 26 (80%) in Group B.

As time progressed and more research was conducted, nebulized forms of amikacin began to replace its IV form when it was found that repeated doses of aerosolized amikacin could be safely administered and bring about improvement in mechanically ventilated patients without causing serious side effects or increasing mortality. A study was conducted that involved administering aerosol amikacin administered with IV treatment in ventilated patients who acquired gram-negative pneumonia. Patients were randomized where one group received aerosolized amikacin daily with placebo (normal saline) 12 hours later, one received amikacin twice daily, and the other placebo twice daily [43]. The results revealed that the mean number of IV antibiotics were two times greater with placebo than with twice-daily amikacin ($P < 0.02$). For daily and twice-daily amikacin, the serum Cmax were 1.3 and 1.8 μg/ml, respectively, on day 1, and 2.3 and 3.2 μg/ml on day 3. Mean trough levels were 0.87 and 1.49 μg/ml. Tracheal aspirate levels (mean) on day 3 were found to be 6.9 mg/ml (daily) and 16.2 mg/ml (twice daily). This shows that mechanically ventilated patients with gram-negative pneumonia can safely be treated with repeated doses of adjunctive inhaled amikacin as it is well tolerated by most while simultaneously lessening the need for frequent IV antibiotic use.

Recent study done by Lu et al. proves that nebulized form of amikacin works best against intermediate strains and reduces chances of developing antibiotic resistance. In this study, 40 patients with ventilator-associated pneumonia caused by *Pseudomonas aeruginosa* were studied in a comparative phase II trial. Twenty patients infected with susceptible or intermediate strains were treated with nebulized ceftazidime and amikacin (25 $mg{\cdot}kg^{-1}{\cdot}d^{-1}$). Seventeen patients infected with susceptible strains received intravenous ceftazidime and amikacin (15 $mg{\cdot}kg^{-1}{\cdot}d^{-1}$). After 8 days of treatment, acquisition of antibiotic resistance was seen exclusively in the intravenous group. Moreover, in the aerosol group, four patients infected with intermediate strains were treated successfully [44].

Furthermore, it has also been seen that if administered via inhalation prophylactically within the right time frame, amikacin has shown to reduce chances of development of VAP in the first place. A study enrolled 850 patients who underwent randomization to have 417 placed in the amikacin group and 430 in the placebo group. Amikacin nebulizations were administered thrice daily at a dose of 20 mg/kg in 337 patients (81%) in the amikacin for 28 days. The results showed that ventilator-associated pneumonia developed in 62 patients (15%) in the amikacin group and in 95 patients (22%) in the placebo group, with a difference in mean survival time to ventilator-associated pneumonia of 1.5 days, 95% confidence interval [CI]of 0.6 to 2.5, and $P = 0.004$. Similarly, 74 patients (18%) in the amikacin group developed infection-related ventilator-associated complication, while 111 patients (26%) in the placebo group developed similar complications (hazard ratio, 0.66; 95% CI, 0.50 to 0.89), proving that inhaled amikacin can reduce the burden of ventilator-associated pneumonia in ICU patients [45].

3.5 Prevention of VAP

With better understanding of the pathophysiology of VAP, new advancements have been made for the prevention of VAP. These include non-pharmacological as well as pharmacological interventions.

4. Non-pharmacological preventative strategies

4.1 Utilization of preventative bundles

Preventative bundles, consisting of evidence-based preventive measures, are implemented to maximize efficacy. Although challenging to procure and implement due to the necessity of continuous surveillance to ensure compliance and measure improvements, several studies have proven their effectiveness in reducing the occurrence of VAP. For instance, in one study, the incidence of VAP decreased from 8.6 per 1000 ventilator days before bundle implementation to 2.0 per 1000 ventilator days after ($P < 0.001$) [46]. Similar studies have reported comparable results.

4.2 Modification of artificial airways

Efforts have been made to improve the design of endotracheal tubes (ETTs) to enhance sealing properties. For instance, researchers found that the ratio between the diameter of the cuff and the tracheal internal lumen, cuff length, and cuff pressures were associated with tracheal sealing (Li Bassi et al.) [47]. Additionally, subglottic secretion suction (SSS) has shown consistent evidence of benefits in reducing VAP incidence (Mao et al.) [48]. Meta-analyses have confirmed that SSS is associated with a decrease in VAP incidence, decreased ventilator days, and ICU length of stay. A new ETT, the PneuX, has been evaluated in clinical settings, featuring a low-volume, low-pressure silicone cuff and a continuous tracheal seal monitor system [4].

4.3 Adjustment of body position

Studies have demonstrated that semi-recumbent positions with higher head-of-the-bed orientation reduce the risk of clinically suspected VAP compared to supine positions. Moderate quality evidence supports this finding [49].

5. Pharmacological preventative strategies

5.1 Oropharyngeal decontamination

Decontamination agents such as chlorhexidine and hydrogen peroxide have been widely successful in preventing VAP, as oral hygiene plays a significant role in the development of respiratory infections. High-quality evidence supports the efficacy of chlorhexidine in reducing the incidence of VAP compared to placebo or usual care. Similarly, hydrogen peroxide has shown significant effectiveness in reducing VAP incidence [50].

5.2 Prophylactic antimicrobials

Antimicrobials administered intravenously, nebulized, or to the gastrointestinal tract have been used to prevent VAP. However, concerns about antibiotic resistance arise in the time of multidrug resistance. Studies have shown a lower incidence of gram-negative bacilli and multidrug-resistant bacteria VAP in patients who received colistin, but the long-term deleterious effects of antibiotic resistance require further evidence [51].

5.3 Probiotics

Probiotics, microorganisms administered as individual strains or combinations, have shown promise in reducing VAP incidence. A 2016 meta-analysis supports their use as a preventive strategy to maintain gastrointestinal homeostasis and inhibit colonization [52]. However, larger randomized trials are needed to conclusively establish their benefits.

6. Implications

Despite showing good response to eradicating gram-negative bacilli in ventilated patients, numerous studies have revealed why treatment with amikacin might not be sufficient. One of the biggest reasons for this is antibiotic resistance. Studies from as early as the 1980s have documented the development of resistance to amikacin, along with multiple other antimicrobials [53]. Resistance can develop due to several reasons such as alteration of the target site, enzymatic inactivation of the drug, or establishment of a permeability barrier to the drug [54]. Another common risk factor found to cause amikacin resistance was insufficient dosage and frequently changing medications and doses. Since then, hospitals globally have been taking necessary precautions to prevent or at least slow down the rate at which resistance is developing. This is done by restricting treatment to one antimicrobial at a time and ensuring it is administered at the right dosage [55].

As mentioned earlier, aminoglycosides like amikacin are often paired with other antimicrobials to broaden the antibacterial spectrum and reduce chances of resistance. However, combination therapy with amikacin was found to result in a significantly higher incidence of adverse effects, most noteworthy one being nephrotoxicity [3].

As the fields of medicine and pharmacology are ever evolving to continuously improve quality of care provided to patients and combat restrictions, alternative combination therapies have been found to show better responses to treating VAP by reducing ICU mortality, decreasing duration of mechanical ventilation, and lessening duration of ICU stay while being a lot more cost effective. Furthermore, these new medications also produce lesser side effects than combination treatments with amikacin [6].

In addition to these recent advancements, a recent study found that nebulized amikacin might not have a major role to play in treating VAP. When compared with a placebo, it was found that there was no particular difference in survival rates of either groups: 191 (75%) patients in the Amikacin Inhale group survived compared to 196 (77%) patients in the placebo group (odds ratio 0·841, 95% CI 0·554–1·277; $p = 0{\cdot}43$), further raising doubts about the active and significant role of inhaled amikacin with intravenous antibiotic treatment in mechanically ventilated patients who have acquired gram-negative VAP [1].

Nevertheless, despite aminoglycosides being an older group of antibiotics, they continue to be clinically valuable, particularly amikacin for its broad-spectrum bactericidal activity especially against gram-negative bacteria if used correctly with adequate monitoring, dosing, and administration timings to reduce development of side effects and resistance.

7. Conclusion

Based on current research, amikacin has proven successful in treating ventilator-associated pneumonia with minimal adverse effects such as nephrotoxicity and has markedly reduced the duration of mechanical ventilation and ICU stay. Its nebulized form demonstrates the most effective response against intermediate strains and has also been used prophylactically in the prevention of VAP. Utilization of the aforementioned preventative, diagnostic, and therapeutic recommendations may allow for improved outcomes seen in mechanically ventilated patients suffering from ventilator-associated pneumonia.

Author details

Abdul Moeed[1*], Zoha Bilal[2], Fizzah Batool[1], Asma Batool Zaidi[3], Muhammad Arsalan Jamil[4] and Salim Surani[5]

1 Dow Medical College, Karachi, Pakistan

2 Aga Khan University, Karachi, Pakistan

3 Dow University Hospital Ojha, Karachi, Pakistan

4 Department of Anaesthesiology, Civil Hospital Karachi, Pakistan

5 Texas A&M University, College Station, Texas, USA

*Address all correspondence to: abdulmoeed117@outlook.com

References

[1] Klompas M. Ventilator-associated events: What they are and what they are not. Respiratory Care. 2019;**64**(8):953-961. DOI: 10.4187/respcare.07059

[2] Song X, Chen Y, Li X. Differences in incidence and outcome of ventilator-associated pneumonia in surgical and medical ICUs in a tertiary hospital in China. Clinical Respiratory Journal. 2014;**8**(3):262-268. DOI: 10.1111/crj.12036

[3] Koenig SM, Truwit JD. Ventilator-associated pneumonia: Diagnosis, treatment, and prevention. Clinical Microbiology Reviews. 2006;**19**(4):637-657. DOI: 10.1128/CMR.00051-05

[4] Bassi GL, Senussi T, Xiol EA. Prevention of ventilator-associated pneumonia. Current Opinion in Infectious Diseases. 2017;**30**(2):214-220. DOI: 10.1097/QCO.0000000000000358

[5] Torres A, Niederman MS, Chastre J, Ewig S, Fernandez-Vandellos P, Hanberger H, et al. International ERS/ESICM/ESCMID/ALAT guidelines for the management of hospital-acquired pneumonia and ventilator-associated pneumonia: Guidelines for the management of hospital-acquired pneumonia (HAP)/ventilator-associated pneumonia (VAP) of the European Respiratory Society (ERS), European Society of Intensive Care Medicine (ESICM), European Society of Clinical Microbiology and Infectious Diseases (ESCMID) and Asociación Latinoamericana del Tórax (ALAT). The European Respiratory Journal. 2017;**50**(3):1700582. DOI: 10.1183/13993003.00582-2017

[6] Chlebicki MP, Safdar N. Topical chlorhexidine for prevention of ventilator-associated pneumonia: A meta-analysis. Critical Care Medicine. 2007;**35**(2):595-602. DOI: 10.1097/01.CCM.0000253395.70708.AC

[7] DeLong PA, Kotloff RM. An overview of pulmonary host defense. Seminars in Roentgenology. 2000;**35**(2):118-123. DOI: 10.1053/ro.2000.6150

[8] Karvouniaris M, Makris D, Zygoulis P, Triantaris A, Xitsas S, Mantzarlis K, et al. Nebulised colistin for ventilator-associated pneumonia prevention. The European Respiratory Journal. 2015;**46**(6):1732-1739. DOI: 10.1183/13993003.02235-2014

[9] Iregui M, Ward S, Sherman G, Fraser VJ, Kollef MH. Clinical importance of delays in the initiation of appropriate antibiotic treatment for ventilator-associated pneumonia. Chest. 2002;**122**(1):262-268. DOI: 10.1378/chest.122.1.262

[10] Dubois, VArpin C, Melon M, Melon B, Andre C, Frigo C, Quentin C. Nosocomial outbreak due to a multiresistant strain of Pseudomonas aeruginosa P12: Efficacy of Cefepime-amikacin therapy and analysis of β-lactam resistance. Journal of Clinical Microbiology. 2001;**39**:2072-2078. DOI: 10.1128/jcm.39.6.2072-2078.2001

[11] Rea-Neto A, Youssef NC, Tuche F, Brunkhorst F, Ranieri VM, Reinhart K, et al. Diagnosis of ventilator-associated pneumonia: A systematic review of the literature. Critical Care. 2008;**12**(2):R56. DOI: 10.1186/cc6877 Epub 2008 Apr 21

[12] Pham TN, Neff MJ, Simmons JM, Gibran NS, Heimbach DM, Klein MB. The clinical pulmonary infection score poorly predicts pneumonia in

patients with burns. Journal of Burn Care & Research. 2007;**28**(1):76-79. DOI: 10.1097/BCR.0b013E31802C88DB

[13] American Thoracic Society; Infectious Diseases Society of America. Guidelines for the management of adults with hospital-acquired, ventilator-associated, and healthcare-associated pneumonia. American Journal of Respiratory and Critical Care Medicine. 2005;**171**(4):388-416. DOI: 10.1164/rccm.200405-644ST

[14] Papazian L, Thomas P, Garbe L, Guignon I, Thirion X, Charrel J, et al. Bronchoscopic or blind sampling techniques for the diagnosis of ventilator-associated pneumonia. American Journal of Respiratory and Critical Care Medicine. 1995;**152**(6 Pt. 1):1982-1991. DOI: 10.1164/ajrccm.152.6.8520766

[15] Gupta D, Agarwal R, Aggarwal AN, Singh N, Mishra N, Khilnani GC, et al. Guidelines for diagnosis and management of community- and hospital-acquired pneumonia in adults: Joint ICS/NCCP(I) recommendations. Lung India. 2012;**29**(Suppl. 2):S27-S62. DOI: 10.4103/0970-2113.99248

[16] Li HY, Wang HS, Wang YL, Wang J, Huo XC, Zhao Q. Management of ventilator-associated pneumonia: Quality assessment of clinical practice guidelines and variations in recommendations on drug therapy for prevention and treatment. Frontiers in Pharmacology. 2022;**13**:903378. DOI: 10.3389/fphar.2022.903378

[17] Pugin J, Auckenthaler R, Mili N, Janssens JP, Lew PD, Suter PM. Diagnosis of ventilator-associated pneumonia by bacteriologic analysis of bronchoscopic and nonbronchoscopic "blind" bronchoalveolar lavage fluid. The American Review of Respiratory Disease. 1991;**143**(5 Pt. 1):1121-1129. DOI: 10.1164/ajrccm/143.5_Pt_1.1121

[18] Kalil AC, Metersky ML, Klompas M, Muscedere J, Sweeney DA, Palmer LB, et al. Management of Adults with Hospital-acquired and Ventilator-associated Pneumonia: 2016 clinical practice guidelines by the Infectious Diseases Society of America and the American Thoracic Society. Clinical Infectious Diseases. 2016;**63**(5):e61-e111. DOI: 10.1093/cid/ciw353. Epub 2016 Jul 14. [Erratum in: Clin Infect Dis. 2017 May 1;64(9):1298. Erratum in: Clin Infect Dis. 2017 Oct 15;65(8):1435. Erratum in: Clin Infect Dis. 2017 Nov 29;65(12):2161]

[19] Association SoCRDoCM. Guidelines for atomization treatment of patients with mechanical ventilation. Chinese Journal of Critical Care Medicine. 2021;**7**(03):193-203. DOI: 10.3877/cma.j.issn.2096-1537.2021.03.001

[20] Infectious disease group RmboCMA. Guidelines for diagnosis and treatment of adult HAP and VAP in China. The Chinese Journal of Tuberculosis and Respiratory Diseases. 2018;**41**(4):255-280. DOI: 10.3760/cma.j.issn.1001-09392018.04.006

[21] Kalil AC, Metersky ML, Klompas M, Muscedere J, Sweeney DA, Palmer LB, et al. Executive summary: Management of Adults with Hospital-acquired and Ventilator-associated Pneumonia: 2016 clinical practice guidelines by the Infectious Diseases Society of America and the American Thoracic Society. Clinical Infectious Diseases. 2016;**63**(5):575-582. DOI: 10.1093/cid/ciw504. Erratum In: Clinical Infectious Diseases. 1 May 2017;**64**(9):1298. Erratum In: Clinical Infectious Diseases. 1 Oct 2017;**65**(7):1251. PMID: 27521441; PMCID: PMC4981763

[22] Shi Y, Huang Y, Zhang TT, Cao B, Wang H, Zhuo C, et al. Chinese guidelines for the diagnosis and treatment of hospital-acquired pneumonia and

ventilator-associated pneumonia in adults (2018 edition). Journal of Thoracic Disease. 2019;**11**(6):2581-2616. DOI: 10.21037/jtd.2019.06.09

[23] Chou CC, Shen CF, Chen SJ, Chen HM, Wang YC, Chang WS, et al. Infectious Diseases Society of Taiwan. Taiwan Society of Pulmonary and Critical Care Medicine; Medical Foundation in Memory of Dr. Deh-Lin Cheng; Foundation of Professor Wei-Chuan Hsieh for Infectious Diseases Research and Education; CY Lee's Research Foundation for Pediatric Infectious Diseases and Vaccines; 4th Guidelines Recommendations for Evidence-based Antimicrobial agents use in Taiwan (GREAT) Working Group. Recommendations and guidelines for the treatment of pneumonia in Taiwan. Journal of Microbiology, Immunology, and Infection. 2019;**52**(1):172-199. DOI: 10.1016/j.jmii.2018.11.004. Epub 2018 Dec 6

[24] Mikasa K, Aoki N, Aoki Y, Abe S, Iwata S, Ouchi K, et al. JAID/JSC guidelines for the treatment of respiratory infectious diseases: The Japanese Association for Infectious Diseases/Japanese Society of Chemotherapy - the JAID/JSC guide to clinical Management of Infectious Disease/guideline-preparing committee respiratory infectious disease WG. Journal of Infection and Chemotherapy. 2016;**22**(7 Suppl):S1-S65. DOI: 10.1016/j.jiac.2015.12.019. Epub 2016 Jun 15

[25] Leone M, Bouadma L, Bouhemad B, Brissaud O, Dauger S, Gibot S, et al. Hospital-acquired pneumonia in ICU. Anaesth Crit Care Pain Med. 2018;**37**(1):83-98. DOI: 10.1016/j.accpm.2017.11.006. Epub 2017 Nov 15

[26] Rodríguez-Pardo D, Escolà-Vergé L, Sellarès-Nadal J, Corona PS, Almirante B, Pigrau C. Periprosthetic joint infection prophylaxis in the elderly after hip Hemiarthroplasty in proximal femur fractures: Insights and challenges. Antibiotics (Basel). 2021;**10**(4):429. DOI: 10.3390/antibiotics10040429

[27] Goodlet KJ, Nicolau DP, Nailor MD. In vitro comparison of Ceftolozane-Tazobactam to traditional Beta-lactams and Ceftolozane-Tazobactam as an alternative to combination antimicrobial therapy for Pseudomonas aeruginosa. Antimicrobial Agents and Chemotherapy. 2017;**61**(12):e01350-e01317. DOI: 10.1128/AAC.01350-17

[28] Bassetti M, Castaldo N, Cattelan A, Mussini C, Righi E, Tascini C, et al. Ceftolozane/tazobactam for the treatment of serious Pseudomonas aeruginosa infections: A multicentre nationwide clinical experience. International Journal of Antimicrobial Agents. 2019;**53**(4):408-415. DOI: 10.1016/j.ijantimicag.2018.11.001. Epub 2018 Nov 8

[29] Bassetti M, Mularoni A, Giacobbe DR, Castaldo N, Vena A. New antibiotics for hospital-acquired pneumonia and ventilator-associated pneumonia. Seminars in Respiratory and Critical Care Medicine. 2022;**43**(2):280-294. DOI: 10.1055/s-0041-1740605. Epub 2022 Jan 27

[30] Novelli A, Del Giacomo P, Rossolini GM, Tumbarello M. Meropenem/vaborbactam: A next generation β-lactam β-lactamase inhibitor combination. Expert Review of Anti-Infective Therapy. 2020;**18**(7):643-655. DOI: 10.1080/14787210.2020.1756775. Epub 2020 May 3

[31] Shorttidge D, Deshpande LM, Duncan LR, Streit JM, Castanheira M. 1590.ActivityofMeropenem-Vaborbactam and single-agent comparators against Enterobacterales isolates including

KPC-producing isolates, from European patients hospitalized with pneumonia including ventilator-associated pneumonia (2014-2019). Open Forum Infectious Diseases. 2020;7(Supplement_1):S792. DOI: 10.1093/ofid/ofaa439.1770

[32] Lob SH, Hackel MA, Kazmierczak KM, Young K, Motyl MR, Karlowsky JA, et al. In vitro activity of Imipenem-Relebactam against gram-negative ESKAPE pathogens isolated by clinical Laboratories in the United States in 2015 (results from the SMART global surveillance program). Antimicrobial Agents and Chemotherapy. 2017;**61**(6):e02209-e02216. DOI: 10.1128/AAC.02209-16

[33] Sellarès-Nadal J, Eremiev S, Burgos J, Almirante B. An overview of cilastatin + imipenem + relebactam as a therapeutic option for hospital-acquired and ventilator-associated bacterial pneumonia: Evidence to date. Expert Opinion on Pharmacotherapy. 2021;**22**(12):1521-1531. DOI: 10.1080/14656566.2021.1939680. Epub 2021 Jul 12

[34] Bassetti M, Echols R, Matsunaga Y, Ariyasu M, Doi Y, Ferrer R, et al. Efficacy and safety of cefiderocol or best available therapy for the treatment of serious infections caused by carbapenem-resistant gram-negative bacteria (CREDIBLE-CR): A randomised, open-label, multicentre, pathogen-focused, descriptive, phase 3 trial. The Lancet Infectious Diseases. 2021;**21**(2):226-240. DOI: 10.1016/S1473-3099(20)30796-9. Epub 2020 Oct 12

[35] Brun-Buisson C, Sollet JP, Schweich H, Brière S, Petit C, for the VAP Study Group. Treatment of ventilator-associated pneumonia with piperacillin-Tazobactam/amikacin versus Ceftazidime/amikacin: A Multicenter. Randomized Controlled Trial, Clinical Infectious Diseases. 1998;**26**(2):346-354. DOI: 10.1086/516294

[36] Pien FD, Ho PWL. Antimicrobial spectrum, pharmacology, adverse effects, and therapeutic use of amikacin sulfate. American Journal of Hospital Pharmacy. 1981;**38**(7):981-989. DOI: 10.1093/ajhp/38.7.981

[37] Block M, Blanchard DL. Aminoglycosides. In: StatPearls. Treasure Island (FL): StatPearls Publishing; 17 July 2023

[38] Ahmed AM, Abdalla W. Effect of extended infusion of meropenem and nebulized amikacin on gram-negative multidrug-resistant ventilator-associated pneumonia. Saudi Journal of Anaesthesia. 2018;**12**(1):89-94. DOI: 10.4103/sja.SJA_148_17

[39] Schreiber AF, Arana H, Lu X, Aubry A, Lv J, Rouby J-J, et al. Late-breaking abstract: Nebulized intravenous amikacin in ventilator-associated pneumonia caused by pseudomonas aeruginosa; European Respiratory Journal [Internet]. 1 Sep 2016;**48**(suppl 60):PA363. Available from: http://erj.ersjournals.com/content/48/suppl_60/PA363.abstract

[40] El Fawy DM, Ibrahim AY, Abdulmageed AMM, et al. A comparative study between effect of combined intravenous and nebulized amikacin versus intravenous amikacin alone in mechanically ventilated patients with ventilator-associated pneumonia (VAP). Ain-Shams Journal of Anesthesiology. 2020;**12**:47. DOI: 10.1186/s42077-020-00098-3

[41] Niederman M, Chastre J, Corkery K, et al. Decrease in intravenous antibiotic use with adjunctive aerosolized amikacin treatment in intubated mechanically

ventilated patients with gram-negative pneumonia. Critical Care. 2007;**11**(Suppl. 2):P97. DOI: 10.1186/cc5257

[42] Lu Q et al. Nebulized ceftazidime and amikacin in ventilator-associated pneumonia caused by Pseudomonas aeruginosa. American Journal of Respiratory and Critical Care Medicine. 2011;**184**(1):106-115. DOI: 10.1164/rccm.201011-1894OC

[43] Ehrmann S et al. Inhaled amikacin to prevent ventilator-associated pneumonia. The New England Journal of Medicine. 2023;**389**(22):2052-2062. DOI: 10.1056/NEJMoa2310307

[44] Wormser GP, Tatz J, Donath J. Endemic resistance to amikacin among hospital isolates of gram-negative bacilli: Implications for therapy. Infection Control. 1983;**4**(2):93-99

[45] Acar JF, Goldstein FW, Menard R, Bleriot J-P. Strategies in aminoglycoside use and impact upon resistance. The American Journal of Medicine. 1986;**80**(6, Supplement 2):82-87. ISSN 0002-9343. DOI: 10.1016/0002-9343(86)90484-5

[46] Batra P, Mathur P, John NV, Nair SA, Aggarwal R, Soni KD, et al. Impact of multifaceted preventive measures on ventilator-associated pneumonia at a single surgical Centre. Intensive Care Medicine. 2015;**41**(12):2231-2232. DOI: 10.1007/s00134-015-4047-z

[47] Li Bassi G, Ranzani OT, Marti JD, Giunta V, Luque N, Isetta V, et al. An in vitro study to assess determinant features associated with fluid sealing in the design of endotracheal tube cuffs and exerted tracheal pressures. Critical Care Medicine. 2013;**41**(2):518-526. DOI: 10.1097/CCM.0b013e31826a4804

[48] Mao Z, Gao L, Wang G, Liu C, Zhao Y, Gu W, et al. Subglottic secretion suction for preventing ventilator-associated pneumonia: An updated meta-analysis and trial sequential analysis. Critical Care (London, England). 2016;**20**(1):353. DOI: 10.1186/s13054-016-1527-7

[49] Wang L, Li X, Yang Z, Tang X, Yuan Q, Deng L, et al. Semi-recumbent position versus supine position for the prevention of ventilator-associated pneumonia in adults requiring mechanical ventilation. The Cochrane Database of Systematic Reviews. 2016;**2016**(1):CD009946. DOI: 10.1002/14651858.CD009946.pub2

[50] Xie X, Lyu J, Hussain T, Li M. Drug prevention and control of ventilator-associated pneumonia. Frontiers in Pharmacology. 2019;**10**:298. DOI: 10.3389/fphar.2019.00298

[51] Manzanares W, Lemieux M, Langlois PL, Wischmeyer PE. Probiotic and synbiotic therapy in critical illness: A systematic review and meta-analysis. Critical Care (London, England). 2016;**19**:262. DOI: 10.1186/s13054-016-1434-y

[52] Nobahar M, Razavi MR, Malek F, Ghorbani R. Effects of hydrogen peroxide mouthwash on preventing ventilator-associated pneumonia in patients admitted to the intensive care unit. The Brazilian Journal of Infectious Diseases : An Official Publication of the Brazilian Society of Infectious Diseases. 2016;**20**(5):444-450. DOI: 10.1016/j.bjid.2016.06.005

[53] Marcus R, Paul M, Elphick H, Leibovici L. Clinical implications of β-lactam–aminoglycoside synergism: Systematic review of randomised trials. International Journal of Antimicrobial Agents, Volume. 2011;**37**(6):491-503. ISSN 0924-8579. DOI: 10.1016/j.ijantimicag.2010.11.029

[54] Moied AS et al. Treatment of ventilator-associated pneumonia with piperacillin-tazobactum and amikacin vs cefepime and levofloxacin: A randomized prospective study. Indian Journal of Critical Care Medicine. 2007;**11**(3):117-121

[55] Niederman MS et al. Inhaled amikacin adjunctive to intravenous standard-of-care antibiotics in mechanically ventilated patients with gram-negative pneumonia (INHALE): A double-blind, randomised, placebo-controlled, phase 3, superiority trial. The Lancet Infectious Diseases. 2020;**20**(3):330-340

Chapter 6

ICU without Borders: We Reached out and MET them

Mainak Majumdar

Abstract

Rapid response systems and MET teams are now recognised as integral components of patient safety measures in health care. While their roles have continued to evolve over the last two decades, most healthcare systems have adopted a model of ICU-led MET teams. We review the current role of ICU-led MET teams within the healthcare ecosystem, including their scope, structure, governance, and contribution to system-wide quality and safety approaches. We also explore the increasing input of rapid response systems into areas of health care not within the traditional remit of intensive care medicine, from end-of- life decision-making to clinical governance, and the increasing reliance of ward-based teams on support from their colleagues in ICU to provide safe, high-quality patient-centric care in modern healthcare systems.

Keywords: rapid response team, rapid response system, medical emergency team, deteriorating patient, patient safety

1. Introduction

Data from many health systems worldwide suggest that 15–20% of hospitalised patients develop serious adverse events [1, 2]. Up to 80% of these adverse events are preceded by physiological and biochemical derangements that can occur over hours and sometimes days [3–5]. Furthermore, many adverse events leading to significant deterioration, including unplanned admissions to intensive care unit (ICU), in-hospital cardiac arrest, and unexpected death, may be due to delays or deficiencies in medical management prior to deterioration, meaning that the majority of these may be preventable [1–2, 6].

Efforts to minimise harm from such incidents and enhance patient safety during hospital admission have become a cornerstone of patient-centric care in healthcare systems worldwide. Beginning with dedicated cardiac arrest teams, solutions to this problem have been in evolution for over two decades now, and varying nomenclatures—Rapid Response Team (RRT), Critical Care Outreach Team (CCOT), and Medical Emergency Team (MET)—are in use in different parts of the world.

Patient deterioration itself is a complex phenomenon and the nature and trajectory of patient deterioration—whether due to natural trajectory of disease, or errors of omission or commission during medical management—is often dependent on the patient population being served by the health service.

Furthermore, there is considerable heterogeneity in personnel, resources, and equipment available to any health service, and this is reflected in the thresholds at which such emergency responses are triggered for patients, the personnel available to provide a meaningful response, and the nature of the response (interventions, outcomes and dispositions). Detailing every possible scenario is outside the scope of this chapter.

In the interests of uniform nomenclature, this chapter will refer to all physiologic deteriorations triggering a health system response as rapid response system (RRS) activations, the responding teams as Medical Emergency Teams (MET team), and primarily consider health services with access to intensive care (ICU) facilities.

2. We reached out and MET

General hospital wards are not staffed or equipped to provide intensive observations and treatments available in critical care areas such as ICU, high dependency units (HDU), emergency departments (ED), or operating theatres (OR). The intent behind rapid-response systems is to identify and respond to patients outside the critical care environment who are at risk of progressing to a serious adverse event such as cardiac arrest, unanticipated ICU admission, or death [7].

2.1 Why have we MET?

Nearly 90% of patients who needed RRS activation were also reviewed by the home teams in the 24 hours preceding this [7]. Interestingly, patients receiving only a home team review prior to RRS were likelier to have higher mortality than if they had a recent ICU review or had recently been discharged from a critical care area [7]. There was little influence of availability of the home team on the likelihood of patients triggering RRS, as evidenced by the day (weekday versus weekend) or time (business hours versus after hours), or on disposition of patients by the MET teams [8, 9].

MET teams and RRS represent an intuitively simple concept: When a patient demonstrates signs of imminent clinical deterioration, a team of providers is summoned to the bedside to immediately assess and treat the patient with the goal of preventing ICU transfer, cardiac arrest, or death. This is a step forward from "cardiac arrest" or "Code Blue" teams, which can only be summoned after cardiopulmonary arrest occurs, with accompanying high mortality and morbidity. MET teams, on the other hand, intervene during the critical period of deterioration on patients in general medical and surgical wards [10].

RRS have become integral to the culture of patient safety in healthcare services across the world. The National Health Service (NHS) in UK has been at the forefront of safety culture in health care. The Royal College of Physicians developed the National Early Warning Score (NEWS) to standardise identification of patients at risk of deterioration in hospital. The Australian Commission on Safety and Quality in Health Care (ACSQHC) determines the National Safety and Quality Health Service Standards (NSQHSS) that all Australian health services must meet for accreditation, of which Standard 8 ("Recognising and Responding to Acute Deterioration Standard") aims to ensure that a person's acute deterioration is recognised promptly and appropriate action is taken [11]. In the United States, the Joint Commission

Centre for Transforming Healthcare, which also focuses on accreditation of healthcare organisations, has incorporated RRS into the National Patient Safety Goals [12]. The worldwide movement has coalesced into the International Society for Rapid Response Systems (ISRRS), a forum where medical, nursing, managerial, and administrative expertise is shared to improve detection and prevention of patient deterioration, with the goal of improving patient safety in hospitals [13].

2.2 Who have we MET?

MET teams respond to RRS activations in patients admitted to a hospital's non-critical care areas. Thus, the patient population encountered in RRS is reflective of the inpatient population, which can vary between health services.

Physiologic thresholds for RRS activation, too, are reflective of the variations in populations of inpatients. An interesting result has been guidance received by ward teams when recording physiologic observations of their patients using (usually colour-coded) "track and trigger" charts (electronic or paper-based), prompting ward nursing staff to activate RRS as per local protocol (e.g. "Between the Flags" observation charts used in New South Wales and "Observation Recording Charts" used in Victoria, Australia) once critical physiologic thresholds are breached. Electronic records further facilitate calculation of early warning scores such as the National Early Warning Score, version 2 (NEWS2) in the National Health Service (NHS) Trusts in UK, the Modified Early Warning Score (MEWS), and the Canadian Hamilton Early Warning Score (HEWS).

Track and trigger charts have further been refined for specific patient subsets, e.g. The age-specific Victorian Children's Tool for Observation and Response (VicTOR) charts introduced by the Royal Children's Hospital in Melbourne, Australia, to record paediatric vital signs and the Maternity Observations Recording Chart (M-ORC) widely used in Victoria, Australia, to detect deterioration in obstetric patients.

Patients needing RRS activation represent a very small fraction of patients admitted to hospital. However, they represent disproportionately higher resource use, with increased length of stay, high likelihood of unplanned ICU interventions, and greater odds of poorer (death or ongoing care) outcomes (OR 5.5) compared to patients admitted to hospital with similar diagnoses. Hospital mortality increases significantly after the age of 50 and rises rapidly for every decade in age [8, 14]. In-hospital mortality rates as high as 15% (for patients with no limitations on therapy) to 50% (for patients with limitations on care) have been quoted [15].

2.3 What is different now we have MET?

While initial smaller studies [16, 17] indicated that introduction of RRS and MET teams could reduce incidence of unexpected cardiac arrests and hospital mortality, larger multicentre studies like MERIT [18] and subsequent systematic reviews have failed to corroborate this effect [19, 20].

Rapid response systems have come to exemplify the tension between those arguing for swift implementation of conceptually attractive patient safety interventions supported by anecdotal evidence of benefit and those advocating a more rigorous, evidence-based, and inevitably slower, approach [10].

Despite failure to demonstrate direct reduction in unexpected hospital mortality, "before and after" studies support the notion that RRS is of benefit through improvements in multiple surrogate measures—respiratory failure, stroke, severe, sepsis, acute renal failure needing renal replacement, unplanned ICU admissions, perioperative deaths, and postoperative LOS in hospital [21]. There has also been a sustained and progressive reduction in the number of in-hospital cardiac arrests [22], which, in themselves, are a major cause of unexpected in-hospital mortality.

While the MERIT study and multiple subsequent studies [8, 18, 23–25] did demonstrate a significant increase in RRS activations in every health service where such systems have been introduced, one of the significant benefits has been a marked increase in support and uptake by nursing staff. The advantages from this cultural change within the healthcare system are difficult to quantify, but sustained focus on patient safety through early detection and escalation of patient deterioration can only be considered beneficial [25, 26].

About 20% RRS calls occur in patients with pre-existing end-of-life issues and another 10% identify end-of-life issues at the MET [15]. It is unclear whether identification of patients at end-of-life or with significant deterioration at end-of-life through RRS has made any material difference to care delivery at end-of-life [9].

2.4 How soon should we have MET?

About a quarter of RRS activations occur within 24 hours of admission to hospital [27, 28]. ED patients admitted with respiratory conditions, myocardial infarction, or sepsis are at modestly increased risk for unplanned ICU transfer. While they may benefit from better triage from the ED, earlier intervention, or closer monitoring to prevent acute decompensation [29], decisions to discharge from ED to the ward are often made under time constraints based on clinical acumen alone rather than evidence-based guidelines [30]. While these may reflect suboptimal triage before ward transfer, the associated mortality is low [8, 28].

In contrast, RRS activations later in the course of the hospital admission are associated with high mortality [28]. Having the first RRS activation more than 24 hours of admission to hospital is an independent predictor of both increased hospital mortality and length of stay [8]. Initial RRS activation after 48 hours of hospital admission is associated with significantly higher risk of in hospital mortality (OR 1.47) compared to MET calls within 24 hours of admission [8]. Whether these represent disease progression, failure to respond to therapy, suboptimal end-of-life planning, or nosocomial complications is poorly understood.

2.5 We MET again!

Recurrent clinical deterioration and repeat medical emergency team activation are common and associated with increased risk of subsequent ICU admission, increased hospital length of stay, and increased hospital mortality. It may be possible to identify patients at risk of recurrent clinical deterioration following medical emergency team activation and target interventions to improve patient care [31].

These patients often represent substantial resource use for MET teams, are often frail, and have significant comorbidities. The greater the number of MET calls, the higher the levels of frailty and comorbidities (**Figure 1**) [14]. This may represent inadequate management of clinical problems in the ward or suboptimal end-of-life planning, as many have significant treatment limitations in place at the time of RRS activation.

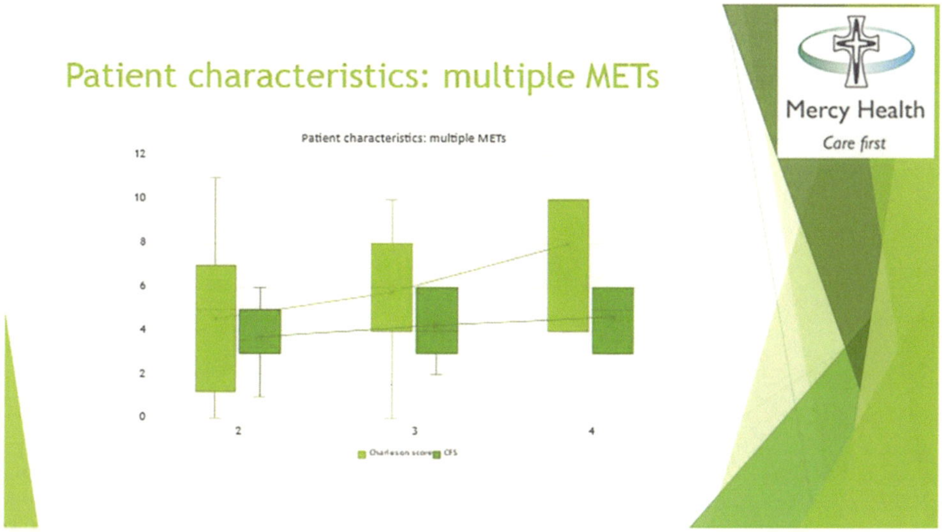

Figure 1.
Box-and-whiskers plot of burden of comorbidities (Charlson score) and frailty (Clinical Frailty Score, CFS) in patients with multiple MET calls. Patients triggering more MET calls have higher comorbidity burden and frailty. (Reproduced with permission from: [14]).

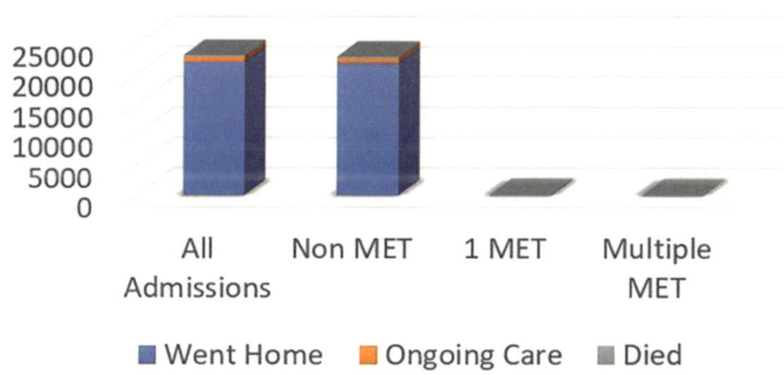

Figure 2.
Death or need for ongoing care after hospital discharge is likelier in the population needing MET calls during the course of their hospital admission. (Reproduced with permission from: [14]).

Figures 2 and **3** [14] demonstrate that while poor outcomes (death or ongoing care) are relatively rare amongst hospital admissions, these outcomes are far likelier in the patients having MET calls. Compared to admissions not associated with RRS, having even one MET call during the admission significantly increases risk of poor outcomes (OR 3.3), while having more than one MET call increases risk of poor outcome substantially beyond this (OR 15.7). In general, having any MET call during an admission increases likelihood of poor outcome (OR 5.5) (**Figure 4**) [14].

MET teams generally triage patients without limitations on medical therapy well [32]. After the second MET call, if escalation of care does not occur, further RRS activations do not significantly change disposition from MET call or hospital outcome (**Figures 4** and **5**) [14].

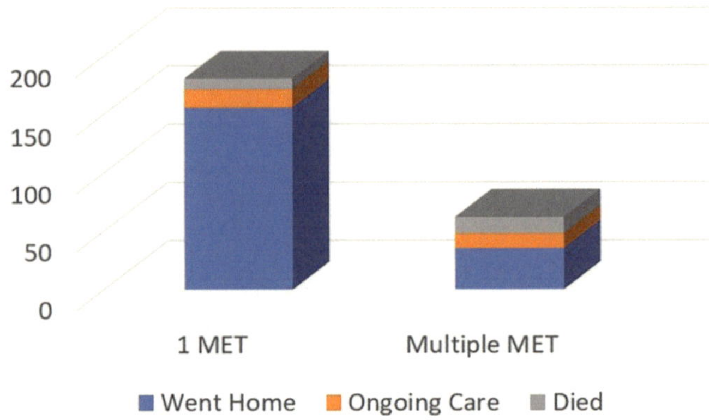

Figure 3.
Likelihood of dying or needing ongoing care is higher in patients needing multiple MET calls than those needing a single MET call. (Reproduced with permission from: [14]).

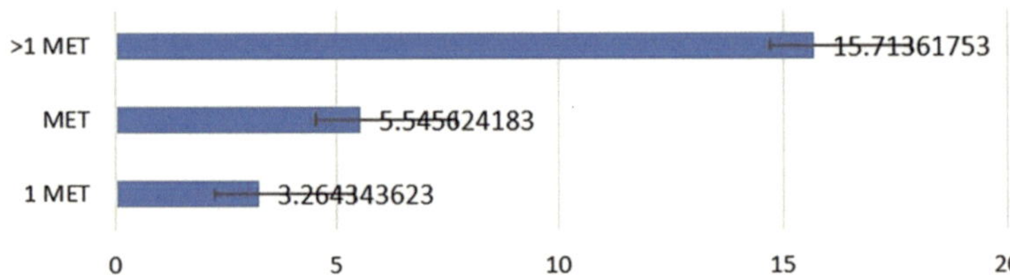

Figure 4.
Patients needing a MET call are likelier to have a poor outcome (death or need for ongoing care) than those who do not (OR5.5). A single MET call increases likelihood of poor outcome (OR3.3) but multiple MET calls increase the risk much more (OR 15.7). (Reproduced with permission from: [14]).

3. Anatomy of a MET system

The minimum standards for ICU-based RRS have been laid out by the College of Intensive Care Medicine of Australia and New Zealand (CICM) [33]. In conjunction with the Joint Position Statement with the Australian and New Zealand Intensive Care Society (ANZICS) [34], it lays the framework for RRS in Australia and New Zealand. Further jurisdictional regulatory requirements for health services, including governance and reporting structures, are laid out by state-wide bodies such as Safer Care Victoria [35] and the Clinical Excellence Commission in New South Wales.

The CICM-ANZICS position acknowledges that there is no clear evidence for the best model for RRS and suggests that the model employed by individual institutions must consider the resources available and the complexity and acuity of the patient mix. Whilst RRS must enhance the ability of all hospital staff to anticipate, identify, and manage patients at risk of deterioration, it may use variable combinations of ward and non-ward-based responders that best meet patient needs and ensure a continuum of patient care. Most hospitals adopt a multi-tiered response and collaborative decision-making between ICU and primary admitting or "home" teams is encouraged. RRS systems working in isolation from home teams are discouraged,

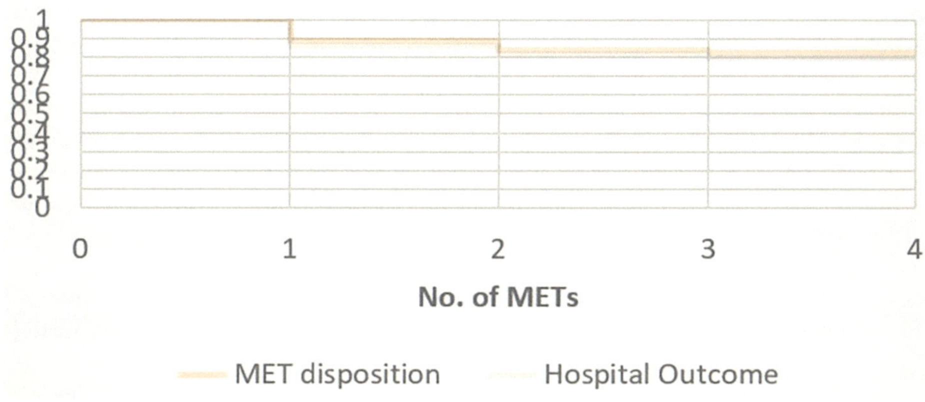

Figure 5.
If escalation does not occur at the 2nd MET call, subsequent RRS calls do not change disposition or hospital outcomes. (Reproduced with permission from: [14]).

as these may conceal underlying systemic contributors to patient deterioration such as staffing levels, inadequate training of ward staff, access to senior medical staff or clinical services, and culture issues resulting in premature or delayed transfer of patients from critical care areas like ED, ICU, and OR to the ward.

In most jurisdictions, RRS is multidisciplinary. It is useful to consider them as comprised of four limbs: (1) an afferent limb, which is the calling criteria and the method of activation, (2) an efferent limb, which is the rapid response team (RRT) itself, (3) an administrative limb, which is responsible for the day-to-day running of the RRS, and (4) the quality improvement and governance limb which addresses system and clinical factors contributing to deterioration.

3.1 The afferent limb

In Victoria, Australia, where RRS activation occurring every 15.9 minutes [35], there is high demand for MET team services.

The optimal set of calling criteria for RRS has not been definitively identified, and there is significant variability in practise between individual institutions, which opt for thresholds and systems to suit their patient populations and staffing. As a general principle, having excessively high thresholds for triggering RRS activations is potentially unsafe for the deteriorating patient and defeats the purpose of RRS activation. While modification of calling criteria, to account for chronic disease and individual patient needs, has also not been validated for safety, there is sound clinical rationale for the practise. It is recommended that modifications to calling criteria for individual patients should involve senior clinicians [34].

Staff involved in RRS are familiar with the A-B-C paradigm in resuscitation, and it may be helpful to consider RRS triggers in the same light, with thresholds individualised to health services to reflect capabilities and inpatient populations.

A. Airway: Impending or actual threat to airway is universally recognised as an emergency in every health system, and it is reasonable to activate RRS for immediate expert assessment and management by an RRS team with airway expertise and equipment.

An occluded airway is frequently followed by cardiorespiratory arrest and is clear grounds for a Code Blue

B. Breathing: Tachypnoea (with or without significant increase in work of breathing) and bradypnea (with or without progressive decrease in respiratory effort) may or may not accompany hypoxia, signified by reduced oxygen saturations (detectable with ward-level monitoring devices like pulse oximeters) or increasing oxygen requirements.

Respiratory distress is often a harbinger of physiologic compromise and comes with approximately doubling (OR 2.05) of risk of in-hospital mortality after MET call [8].

C. Circulation: Tachycardia, symptomatic bradycardia, and new arrhythmias are some of the commonest causes of RRS activation in most healthcare services.

Chest pain in at-risk populations as a symptom of myocardial infarction, pulmonary embolus, or respiratory infection merits immediate attention.

Hypotension has long been recognised as a marker of shock and is also a common trigger for MET calls. Hypertension with malignant symptoms is a significant cause for concern. Hypertension may be of high significance in specific populations like obstetric patients.

Paradoxically, given the traditional focus on cardiovascular parameters for shock, recognition and familiarity with resuscitation protocols often leads to successful resuscitation from cardiovascular compromise prior to progressing to cardiac arrest [8].

D. Disability/altered neurology: Acute alterations in cognition and neurology may not just signify time critical emergencies like stroke or seizures, they may also be early signs of a diverse range of pathologies from sepsis to intoxication, substance withdrawal, delirium, and metabolic encephalopathy. Neurologic emergencies can approximately double (OR 1.83) risk of in-hospital mortality after MET call [8], and, given the diversity of precipitants, early escalation and senior clinician assessments available through RRS activation may be life-saving.

Other/worry-Not every patient deterioration fits neatly into a system-specific paradigm reflected by abnormal vital signs for RRS activation. It has long been recognised that extreme worry by bedside clinical staff merits immediate senior medical review and is grounds for calling the MET team. Recent studies have tried to evaluate and quantify "Worry" in the context of physiologic deterioration of patients [36].

The influence of the indication for MET on in-hospital mortality at a university-linked metropolitan teaching hospital in Australia is shown in **Figure 6** [8].

3.2 The efferent limb

The efferent limb describes the responding clinician team and is often determined by the expertise immediately available. In Australasian hospitals with ICUs,

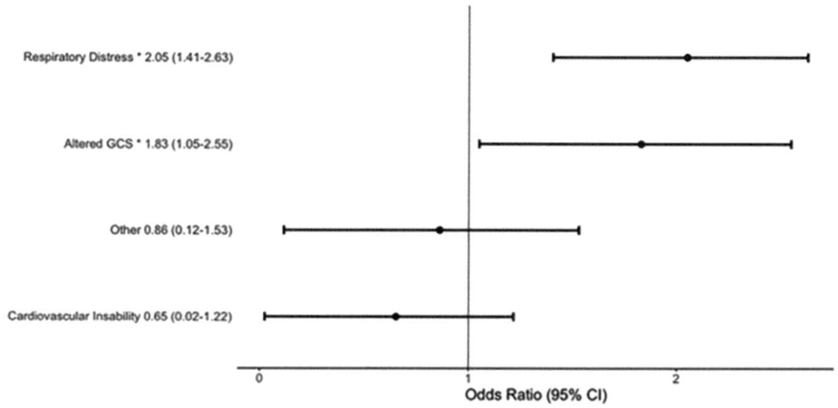

Figure 6.
Odds ratios of death due to various triggers for RRS. Higher chances of dying when the triggers for the RRS were respiratory distress or altered level of consciousness. (Reproduced with permission from: [8]).

it is common for ICU clinical staff to be members of the responding team. In centres without an ICU, the team may be led by either senior nurses, senior medical, or junior medical staff [34]. In North America, hospitalists are increasingly becoming an integral component of RRS, often leading the MET team [10]. The CICM document acknowledges that in hospitals with an ICU, the immediate availability of an ICU team to attend and initiate appropriate life-supportive measures on the ward represents the highest level of patient safety attainable, while recognising that other institution-specific system arrangements may also provide a level of patient safety [33].

The following aspects of the efferent limb are worth considering [33].

1. Staffing: Management of critically ill patients outside the ICU has increasingly become part of ICU core business and is a recognised part of core ICU training. A response time of less than 10 minutes would be typically expected from an ICU team in a large hospital.

   The MET team should be overseen at all times by a specialist in intensive care, immediately available for advice to the ICU RRS responders and to attend to the RRS call where specialist expertise is required.

   While units should ensure attendance of ICU medical staff to RRS calls, "Out of ICU Roles" must not compromise care of the patients within ICU. Trainees and non-specialist medical officers in both ICU and in the RRS teams must have adequate intensivist supervision available at all times.

   All ICU-based RRS should have at least one experienced ICU senior nurse available to attend RRS calls. Their attendance in RRS calls must not compromise nursing care of patients within the ICU.

   Hospitals averaging 2000 or more RRS calls per annum should roster an ICU medical officer and nurse separate to the main ICU treating team exclusively for RRS and have a separate specialist roster for RRS oversight.

The "admitting" team is most familiar with the patient and holds primary responsibility for the patient. This team should have a designated medical officer who is immediately contactable for notification of RRS activation and for involvement in discussions with the ICU MET team members regarding appropriate patient management. Ideally, the afferent limb activation should also alert these doctors about the occurrence of the call in their patient so that they can attend the call in-person.

2. Education: The hospital should have a documented educational program for RRT members.

   The required skill set for ICU staff should focus on knowledge. Technical and non-technical skills and leadership skills should be taught, ideally in the context of immersive team training.

   Success of the RRS requires clinical teams from the RRS and the primary team to work in partnership to ensure timely review and continuity of clinical care. Such an approach has the greatest potential to enhance the skill set of members of each team and ensures that the RRS does not mask organisational problems in the patient's management.

   Education should include the ward-based staff (who are responsible for initiating RRS calls) so both the afferent and efferent limbs of the RRS are effective.

   In hospitals admitting paediatric and obstetric patients, RRT members should undergo specific education in the management of paediatric, neonatal, and obstetric emergencies.

3. Operational requirements: An ICU-based RRS must meet any national criteria set out for such systems.

   An ICU specialist should be nominated as the clinical lead, with appropriate delegated responsibility from the hospital executive providing clinical governance and representing the RRS on relevant hospital committees (e.g. clinical quality, safety, and governance committee), with adequate support from hospital administrative staff employed for quality improvement.

   The clinical lead should meet regularly with nurses and doctors to ensure that the system is running effectively and to resolve problems with the responding team, if any.

   A prospective data collection and evaluation process must be in place and adequately resourced to provide timely and data-driven evaluation of performance that aims to improve the response and outcomes for deteriorating patients.

4. Equipment: The type and quantity of equipment and medications will vary with the type, size, and function of the RRS and must be appropriate to the workload of the MET team as judged by contemporary standards.

There must be a regular system in place for replacement and checking the safety of equipment. Protocols and in-service training for medical and nursing staff need to be available for the use of all equipment, including steps to be taken in the event of malfunction. Portable equipment for mechanical ventilation and monitoring of ventilation, respiratory, and circulatory status must be available for RRS patient transports.

Suggested equipment and medication lists for RRT can be found in the ANZICS and CICM Joint Position Statement on Rapid Response Systems in Australia and New Zealand and the Roles of Intensive Care [34]. Published data suggests RRS efferent limbs in ICU-based systems are good at risk stratification and triage of deteriorating inpatients [32].

3.3 Governance

The governance guidelines from Safer Care Victoria (SCV) [37] concur with CICM and ANZICS guidelines. There are similar principles embedded in other Australasian jurisdictions regarding the establishment of integrated systems, processes, leadership, and culture central to providing safe, effective, accountable, and person-centred care, underpinned by continuous improvement.

At a minimum, RRS must

- Demonstrate compliance with National Safety and Quality Health Service (NSQHS) Standard 8
- Have organisational-level recognition and response governance systems driven by medical lead/s (i.e. heads of unit or equivalent)
- Have clearly defined roles and responsibilities for those involved in the recognition and response system at both organisational and ward level
- Have clear expectations of attending clinician/team accountability within the recognition and response system
- Have clear rapid response escalation policy/policies
- Promote engagement of the attending clinician/team in the recognition and response escalation policies and procedures
- Define organisational clinical indicators for the recognition and response system
- Have a recognition and response system with audit and review processes in place
- Have specific timelines for recognition and response system data collection and data review
- NSQHS Standard 8 (deteriorating patient) committee and/or rapid response team operational lead undertaking risk review and identifies gaps for improvement.

Additional desirable features include

- Hospital executive sponsor to set expectations of engagement
- NSQHS Standard 8 (deteriorating patient) committee including a broad range of multidisciplinary staff
- Standardised process for goals of care/resuscitation planning, including promotion and assistance for patients/families/carers to undertake advanced care planning
- Statewide and national benchmarking of recognition and response systems
- Organisational commitment to recognition and response systems through specific key performance indicators (KPI)
- Support and resource governance staff and clinicians to improve the recognition and response system
- Putting contingency processes, involving attending clinicians/teams in place to guide management of multiple demands on the recognition and response system (e.g. more than one rapid response call occurring at one time)
- Local minimum recognition and response system training requirements
- Ensuring bedside clinicians have adequate assessment skills with regular training updates to maintain skill level
- Development of guidelines for the management of common deterioration syndromes
- Regular multidisciplinary education sessions addressing common deterioration syndromes aimed at bedside clinicians, specific to clinical area.

3.4 Quality and improvement

Communication and feedback between operational, governance, and quality improvement arms of the health service are key for successful implementation of site-specific improvement measures.

RRS involves personnel who do not usually work together assessing and managing the sickest inpatients, often in unfamiliar areas outside of critical care, in a time-critical fashion.

Communication between various elements of RRS, at bedside as well as organisation-wide, is critical for success. At a system level, minimum, communication should include

- Informing patients/families/carers on admission that there is a process for managing deterioration, including a consumer-triggered escalation process
- Open communication and documentation, regarding goals of care, occurs between the patient/family/carer and the attending clinician/team within 48 hours of admission

- Robust rapid response notification system, including notification of attending clinician/team

- Use of crisis management communication skills, such as closed-loop communication, shared mental model, recapping, and graded escalation when escalating and caring for a patient experiencing acute deterioration

- Development of attending clinician/team consultant notification guidelines for when a patient experiences acute deterioration

- Clear, accessible, and open communication with the patient/family/carer regarding patient deterioration and ongoing care from attending clinician/team

- Further review of goals of care, where appropriate, as soon as possible after acute deterioration.

Ideally, communication could also include

- Regular multidisciplinary education and training to support clinicians in the use of crisis management communication skills

  Open discussion and joint decision-making between patient/family/carer, attending clinician/team and rapid response team about ongoing care, especially after repeated RRS activations.

Tiered systems of individual and systemic communication then form the basis of a feedback loop between health consumers, admitting medical staff, ward nursing staff, ICU-based MET team personnel, and organisational staff including personnel in governance, quality improvement, and executive roles. At a bare minimum, the feedback process should

- Be a two-way process that occurs in a "just culture" and focuses on overall improvement of the recognition and response system

- Ensure bedside clinicians are satisfied with the call outcome and plan prior to completion of the RRS

- Ensure debriefing is available post rapid response calls as required

- Ensure clinicians attending the RRS can review performance and system functions, with the aim of system improvement

- Ensure consistent recognition and response system data collection, analysis, and reporting

- Be facilitated by Standard 8 committee/lead, with attending teams clinically reviewing their own rapid response calls to look for patterns and develop strategies for better clinical care

- Ensure individual units and/or wards review their own recognition and response data at morbidity and mortality meetings
- Ensure recognition and response system reports are made available to all clinicians (nursing and medical)
- Ensure feedback to attending clinicians/teams/wards includes recognition and response data and specific trends.

Ideally, feedback should

- Be multidisciplinary (including ward staff) at rapid response morbidity and mortality review sessions
- Involve the attending clinicians/teams involved in audit, review, and feedback of recognition and response systems
- Provide recognition and response system reports are made available to consumers in an accessible way
- Provide transparent, whole of organisation feedback that identifies trends across the health service (i.e. rapid response ground rounds, open access database)
- Have the ability to publicly report rapid response trends and patient outcomes to allow for benchmarking.

4. Conclusions

ICU-based MET teams have become the norm for RRS in hospitals that have ICU on site over the last couple of decades. Models using both ICU medical and nursing staff as primary responders have been successfully introduced.

The commonly accepted model consists of afferent (recognition and escalation at the ward/bedside), efferent (MET teams, often ICU-based, comprising skilled resuscitators with senior decision-making authority and with ability to access more specialised facilities, e.g. ICU), governance (general policy, procedure and oversight of RRS framework as well as jurisdiction and organisation-specific compliance roles), and quality improvement (data gathering, reporting, and benchmarking) arms.

With widespread introduction of RRS, identification and escalation of care to critical care teams at an earlier point in the trajectory of physiologic deterioration means that therapies can be instituted pre-emptively within the general ward setting and only a small proportion of inpatients who trigger an RRS then actually need ICU admission for further management. Measures of patient safety such as unplanned ICU admissions and unexpected cardiac arrests, with attendant high mortality and morbidity, have shown measurable reductions consistently as RRS has become widespread. RRS also provides opportunities to identify patients with significant disease progression, failures to respond to therapy, inadequacies in triage prior to ward transfer, and suboptimal end-of-life planning.

An unavoidable consequence has been the progressive engagement of ICU staff in the governance, organisation, and processes across the remainder of the hospital and in areas not within the traditional remit of ICU medicine. This is a significant change to both care delivery responsibilities and hospital culture. Like all major change, this comes with potential barriers due to entrenched practices and cultures within health systems and these need to be negotiated sensitively and appropriately for the RRS system to successfully provide the intended safety net to patient care in healthcare.

Acknowledgements

The author would like to gratefully acknowledge the work done by the ICU Liaison Nurse Team at Werribee Mercy Hospital for their assistance in data collection and entry and members of the Deteriorating Patient Committee, the organisational governance committee with oversight of the policy and procedure framework relating to NSQHS Standard 8, Mercy Health, Victoria.

Conflict of interest

The author declares no conflict of interest.

Notes/thanks/other declarations

No specific funding was received for this project.

Author details

Mainak Majumdar
Mercy Health, Victoria, Australia

*Address all correspondence to: mmajumdar@mercy.com.au

References

[1] Brennan TA, Leape LL, Laird NM, Hebert L, Localio AR, Lawthers AG. Incidence of adverse events and negligence in hospitalized patients: Results of the Harvard medical practice study. The New England Journal of Medicine. 1991;**324**:370-376

[2] Wilson RM, Runciman WB, Gibberd RW, Harrrison BT, Newby L, Hamilton JD. The quality in Australian health care study. The Medical Journal of Australia. 1995;**163**:458-471

[3] Franklin C, Mathew J. Developing strategies to prevent in-hospital cardiac arrest: Analyzing responses of physicians and nurses in the hours before the event. Critical Care Medicine. 1994;**22**:244-247

[4] Shein RMH, Hazday N, Pena M, Ruben BH, Sprung CL. Clinical antecedents to in-hospital cardiopulmonary arrests. Chest. 1990;**98**:1388-1392

[5] Kause J, Smith G, Prytherch D, Parr M, Flabouris A, Hillman KM. A comparison of antecedents to cardiac arrests, deaths and emergency intensive care admissions in Australia and New Zealand, and the United Kingdom: The ACADEMIA study. Resuscitation. 2004;**62**:275-282

[6] Wilson RM, Harrison BT, Gibberd RW, Hamilton JD. An analysis of the causes of adverse events from the quality in Australian health care study. The Medical Journal of Australia. 1999;**170**:411-415

[7] Trinkle RM, Flabouris A. Medical reviews before cardiac arrest, medical emergency call or unanticipated intensive care unit admission: Their nature and impact on patient outcome. Critical Care and Resuscitation. 2011;**13**:175-180

[8] Majumdar M, Saka E, Kadam U. Is it too soon? We only just MET. In: 18th Emirates Critical Care Conference; Dubai, UAE. 2022

[9] Mullins CF, Psirides A. Activities of a medical emergency team: A prospective observational study of 795 calls. Anaesthesia and Intensive Care. 2016;**44**(1):34-43

[10] Rapid Response Systems. Available from: https://psnet.ahrq.gov/primer/rapid-response-ststems [Accessed: March 26, 2024]

[11] Recognising and Responding to Acute Deterioration Standard. Available from: https://www.safetyandquality.gov.au/standards/nsqhs-standards/recognising-and-responding-acute-deterioration-standard [Accessed: March 26, 2024]

[12] National Patient Safety Goals. Available from: https://psnet.ahrq.gov/issue/national-patient-safety-goals [Accessed: March 26, 2024]

[13] ISRRS Website. Available from: https://rapidresponsesystems.org/ [Accessed: March 27, 2024]

[14] Peng Z, Kaur S, Majumdar M. We have MET before, haven't we? In: Joint ANZICS Safety & Quality and iSRRS Conference; Darwin, Australia. 2023

[15] Jones D. The epidemiology of adult rapid response team patients in Australia. Anaesthesia and Intensive Care. 2014;**42**:213-219

[16] Buist MD, Moore GE, Bernard SA, Waxman BP, Anderson JN, Nguyen TV.

Effects of a medical emergency team on reduction of incidence of and mortality from unexpected cardiac arrests in hospital: Preliminary study. BMJ. 2002;**324**(7334):387-390. DOI: 10.1136/bmj.324.7334.387

[17] Sabahi M, Fanaei SA, Ziaee SA, Falsafi FS. Efficacy of a rapid response team on reducing the incidence and mortality of unexpected cardiac arrests. Trauma Monthly. 2012;**17**(2):270-274. DOI: 10.5812/traumamon.4170. Epub 2012 July 31

[18] MERIT study investigators. Introduction of the medical emergency team (MET) system: A cluster-randomised controlled trial. Lancet. 2005;**365**(9477):2091-2097. DOI: 10.1016/S0140-6736(05)66733-5

[19] Tirkkonen J, Tamminen T, Skrifvars MB. Mortality of rapid response team patients in Australia: A multicentre study. Outcome of adult patients attended by rapid response teams: A systematic review of the literature. Australasian Emergency Care. 2021;**24**(2):112-120. DOI: 10.1016/j.auec.2020.07.008. Epub 2020 September 9

[20] Chan PS, Jain R, Nallmothu BK, et al. Rapid response teams: A systematic review and meta-analysis. Archives of Internal Medicine. 2010;**170**(1):18-26

[21] Bellomo R, Goldsmith D, Uchino S, et al. Prospective controlled trial of effect of medical emergency team on postoperative morbidity and mortality rates. The Medical Journal of Australia. 2003;**179**:283-287

[22] Jones D, Bellomo R, Bates S, et al. Long term effect of a medical emergency team on cardiac arrests in a teaching hospital. Critical Care. 2005;**9**(6):R808-R815. DOI: 10.1186/cc3906. Epub 2005 November

[23] Jones D, Bellomo R. Introduction of a rapid response system: Why we are glad we MET. Critical Care. 2006;**10**:121. DOI: 10.1186/cc4841

[24] Crosbie D, Ghosh A. Medical emergency team (MET) calls at The Northern Hospital (TNH). In: Research Week. Melbourne, Australia: Northern Health; 2020

[25] Cretikos MA, Chen J, Hillman KM. The effectiveness of implementation of the medical emergency team (MET) system and factors associated with use during the MERIT study. Critical Care and Resuscitation. 2007;**9**:205-212

[26] Frawley TJ, Greene K, Majumdar M. Now that we've MET, how do you feel? Evolution of attitudes to rapid response systems across ICU-led and non-ICU-led sites – A multi-site, single institution longitudinal study. In: Joint ANZICS Safety & Quality and iSRRS Conference; Darwin, Australia. 2023

[27] Considine J, Charlesworth D, Currey J. Characteristics and outcomes of patients requiring rapid response system activation within 24 hours of emergency admission. Critical Care and Resuscitation. 2014;**3**(16):184-189

[28] The Medical Emergency Team End-of-life Care Investigators. The timing of rapid-response team activations: A multicentre international study. Critical Care and Resuscitation. 2013;**15**:15-20

[29] Delgado MK, Liu V, Pines JM, et al. Risk factors for unplanned transfer to intensive care within 24 hours of admission from the emergency department in an integrated healthcare system. Journal of Hospital Medicine. 2013;**8**(1):13-19

[30] Calder LA, Arnason T, Vaillancourt C, et al. How do emergency

physicians make discharge decisions? Emergency Medicine Journal. 2015;**32**(9):9-14

[31] Stelfox H, Bagshaw S, Gao S. Characteristics and outcomes for hospitalized patients with recurrent clinical deterioration and repeat medical emergency team activation. Critical Care Medicine. 2014;**42**(7):1601-1609. DOI: 10.1097/CCM.0000000000000315

[32] Schneider A, Warrillow S, Robbins R, et al. An assessment of the triage performance of the efferent arm of the rapid response system. Resuscitation. 2013;**84**(4):477-482

[33] Minimum Standards for Intensive Care Unit-Based Rapid Response Systems (IC-26). Available from: https://cicm.org.au/CICM_Media/CICMSite/Files/Professional/IC-26-Minimum-Standards-for-Intensive-Care-Unit-Based-Rapid-Response-Systems.pdf [Accessed: March 30, 2024]

[34] Joint Position Statement on Rapid Responses Systems in Australia and New Zealand and the Roles of Intensive Care. College Intensive Care Medicine(IC-25). Available from: https://cicm.org.au/CICM_Media/CICMSite/Files/Professional/IC-25-Joint-ANZICS-and-CICM-Rapid-Response-Systems-Position-Statement.pdf [Accessed: March 30, 2024]

[35] Supporting Statewide Medical Emergency Team/Rapid Response. Available from: https://www.safercare.vic.gov.au/best-practice-improvement/improvement-projects/emergency-critical-care/supporting-statewide-medical-emergency-team-rapid-response [Accessed: March 30, 2024]

[36] Haegdorens F, Wils C, Franck E. Predicting patient deterioration by nurse intuition: The development and validation of the nurse intuition patient deterioration scale. International Journal of Nursing Studies. 2023;**142**:104467. DOI: 10.1016/j.ijnurstu.2023.104467

[37] Recognising and Responding to the Deteriorating Patient: Clinical Engagement in Recognition and Response Systems. Available from: https://www.safercare.vic.gov.au/sites/default/files/2020-11/Clinical%20engagement%20in%20recognition%20and%20response%20systems.pdf [Accessed: March 30, 2024]